AMAZING
MEDICAL STORIES

George Burden MD

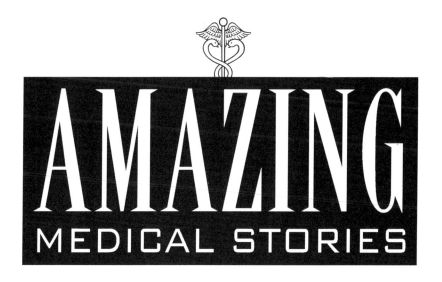

AMAZING
MEDICAL STORIES

George Burden & Dorothy Grant

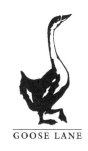

GOOSE LANE

Edited by Sabine Campbell.
Cover illustration "science 19 – Surgeons Operating" by Eyewire.
Cover and interior design by Paul Vienneau.
Printed in Canada by Transcontinental Printing.
10 9 8 7 6 5 4 3 2 1

National Library of Canada Cataloguing in Publication

Burden, George, 1955-
Amazing medical stories / George Burden, Dorothy Grant.

Includes bibliographical references and index.
ISBN 0-86492-347-3

1. Medicine — History — Miscellanea. I. Grant, Dorothy, 1935- II. Title.

R705.B87 2003   610'.9   C2003-900484-8

Published with the financial support of the Canada Council for the Arts,
the Government of Canada through the Book Publishing Industry Development
Program, and the New Brunswick Culture and Sports Secretariat.

Goose Lane Editions
469 King Street
Fredericton, New Brunswick
CANADA E3B 1E5

www.gooselane.com

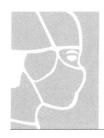

TABLE OF CONTENTS

Introduction 7

Acknowledgements 9

THE DEATH OF THE FRENCH ARMADA 13

ABRAHAM GESNER
   A Doctor Ahead of His Time 17

HENRY MOON
   The Lunar Rogue 23

CATHERINE ANN THOMPSON
   The Silenced Witness 28

ANGUS McASKILL
   A Giant Among Men 35

THE REVEREND JOHN CAMERON
   Diphtheria "Doctor" 39

ANNA SWAN
   The Gentle Giantess 43

DR. DANIEL HALE WILLIAMS
   The First Heart Surgeon 48

THE DOCTOR AND THE KING OF SIAM 53

ALEXANDER GRAHAM BELL
   Medical Inventor 57

THE PHYSICIANS OF THE *TITANIC* 63

A DREADFUL TASK
The Undertakers and the *Titanic* Disaster 71

THE HALIFAX EXPLOSION
Taking Care of the Victims 79

DR. JOHN BRINKLEY
An Infamous Quack 85

DR. ROBERT WRIGHT
Snowmobile Pioneer 91

FERDINAND DEMARA
The Great Impostor 95

DR. R. ARNOLD BURDEN
Springhill Rescuer 101

STEPHEN WEAVER
"Phony Doc Jailed — But Patients Want Him Back" 107

DOCTOR ON THE RUN 114

A TIME TO GRIEVE 118

Further Reading 122

Index 124

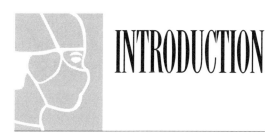

INTRODUCTION

Amazing Medical Stories is a potpourri of true and unusual tales that run the gamut from the tragic to the humorous, from the inspirational to the bizarre. These stories are about great doctors and about charlatans and quacks. They deal with people who pretended to be doctors, with non-physicians who gave important medical gifts, and with medical doctors who gave surprising non-medical gifts to the world. Many take place outside Canada, but all have a link to Canada.

We discovered the treasure trove of Canadian medical history independently. George's training to become a family physician piqued a lively curiosity as to exactly how, medically, we got to where we are today. In the early 1990s, he discovered that Tourette Syndrome may have afflicted the early Roman emperors. Encouraged by Dr. Oliver Sacks, the celebrated American neurologist, and CBC Radio's *Quirks and Quarks*, he next explored the practice of medicine in ancient Egypt. Then, digging into his own country's past, he discovered gold: intriguing stories, unknown to most people, yet begging to be told.

Dorothy's background as a nurse, reporter, and medical society employee infected her with the desire to investigate the mysteries of historical and contemporary medicine. As determined as a medical researcher hell bent on finding a cure for a disease, she relished the detective work, poring over old newspapers and books and tracking down pictures, some more than a hundred years old.

Each of us has published many medical history stories in periodicals, especially *The Medical Post* and *The Halifax Sunday Herald*. Individually, as we wove our stories, we dreamed of gathering them into a book, but it was only when George started to investigate the logistics of actually doing so that we met, first by telephone and then in person. Our shared compulsion to explore and recount the amazing, inspiring, and occasionally very strange stories we had uncovered made us decide to amalgamate our findings in a book to share with others.

We have thoroughly enjoyed the pleasure of finding the captivating tales in *Amazing Medical Stories*. If you'd like to explore these subjects more deeply, we hope you'll be tempted to read some of the articles and books we relished so much; you'll find a list on page 121. We hope that some of our *Amazing Medical Stories* will earn a permanent place in your own repertoire and that you will entertain family and friends with your favourites for years to come.

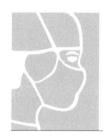

ACKNOWLEDGEMENTS

Many people have helped directly and indirectly with this book, and I am very grateful to them all. I'd especially like to thank Colin Leslie, Leo Charbonneau, Celia Milne and other editors of *The Medical Post*, and Paul O'Connell, of *The Halifax Sunday Herald*, for boosting me into the world of freelance writing. Dr. Jock Murray and the medical writers' group at Dalhousie University have been invaluable in the development of my writing, and I'm also grateful to Dr. Murray and to Dr. Oliver Sacks for their encouragement.

I am grateful to the many individuals and institutions who have given me their help and support, especially Roxanne Leadlay, Aynsley Mac-Farlane and Jess Fraser, Bell Museum, Baddeck, Nova Scotia; Lynn-Marie Richard and the staff of the Maritime Museum of the Atlantic, Halifax; Heather Gillis, Fortress Louisbourg; Frances Lourie, Bridgetown Heritage Society; Regina Mantin, New Brunswick Museum; Val White, *The Medical Post*; and Gary Shutlack, Senior Reference Archivist at the Public Archives of Nova Scotia.

I want to thank the people who have assisted with specific stories, including Dr. Stephen Bedwell, an expert in the ailments of the Duc d'Anville; Dale Swan, great-nephew of Anna Swan, and Dr. Carl Abbott and Dr. Ralph Loebenberg, who helped me to diagnose Swan's final illness; Lorna Johnson, whose references led me to Henry Moon; and the Fundy Geological Museum, Parrsboro, Nova Scotia, which inspired the story about Abraham Gesner. Lois Yorke, Public Archives of Nova Scotia, and journalist Bruce Nunn enabled me to find the descendants of Anna Leonowens, and Dr. Avis Boyar and Thomas Fyshe contributed information and photos of their grandfather. Grant MacDonald helped me with the story about the Reverend John Cameron; Mrs. Ritta Wright and Dr. Robert Wright told me about the mechanical sleigh; and Dr. Arnold Burden provided much information about the Springhill mine disasters. Above all, I am grateful to my wife, Krista Burden, and our family for tolerating Daddy's spending so much time in front of the computer. Thanks also to the staff of Goose Lane Editions for making the dream of my first book a reality. And finally, thanks to Dorothy, my co-author, whose good cheer and sense of humour helped me through the sometimes difficult creative process.

George Burden

While working on *Amazing Medical Stories*, I met some extremely helpful and enthusiastic people, and I wish to express my sincere thanks to those who shared their wisdom. Many librarians and archivists have done exceptional sleuthing on my behalf. I am very grateful to Gary Shutlack, Senior Reference Archivist at the Public Archives of Nova Scotia and an expert on the *Titanic* disaster. The staff at the Keshen Goodman Library, Halifax, were unfailingly helpful, especially Marilyn Baldwin, Ron Bulmer, Gail Tattrie, Denise Vila and Sarah Wenning, as were the reference staff of the Spring Garden Road Library and Patrick Ellis and the staff of the Kellogg Health Sciences Library, Dalhousie University, Halifax. I am also grateful to Arlene Shaner, Reference Librarian, New York Academy of Medicine Library. I offer my sincere thanks to Finn Bower, the Curator of the Shelburne County Museum, and to Dr. Allan Marble and his associates at the Medical History Museum of Nova Scotia Society for their kind help. I owe a special debt of gratitude to my editors, Colin Leslie and Valerie White at *The Medical Post* and Christine Soucie and Claire McIlveen at *The Halifax Sunday Herald*.

I am particularly grateful for the constant and uncomplaining support of my husband, Bill Grant, who continues to be a faithful booster despite the fact that, although we are supposedly retired, my attention is often focused, not on him, but on the computer. For me, co-authoring *Amazing Medical Stories* was a wonderful learning experience. One important lesson was that book publication demands teamwork at its best, and I am grateful to George, an outstanding collaborator. Almost from the moment George and I learned that Goose Lane Editions would publish our book, I realized that I needed the assistance of a league of highly qualified, patient and committed colleagues. I am convinced that my contribution to this book would not have happened without their generous assistance, their patience, and their guidance.

Dorothy Grant

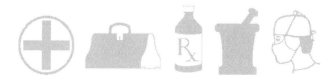

Versions of many of the chapters in *Amazing Medical Stories* have been previously published. Those appearing in *The Medical Post* are: "The Death of Duc D'Anville"; "A Geological MD"; "A Giant Among Men"; "From Preacher to Physician"; "The Giantess of Nova Scotia"; "Dr. Williams: The Greatest Black Surgeon of His Time"; "The Doctors and I"; "Teacher of the Deaf"; "Titanic Doctors Boarded Disaster"; "Master of Deception"; "Digging Up Disaster"; "'Doc' Weaver: Nova Scotia's Physician Imposter"'Doc' Weaver: Nova Scotia's Physician Imposter"; "The Doctor Who Wasn't There"; "Doctor in Profile: A Time to Grieve."

Stories appearing in *The Halifax Sunday Herald* are: "This Officer Was No Gentleman"; "Infamous Dr. Brinkley"; "Pioneer Surgeon"; "'Doc' Weaver: Nova Scotia's Physician Imposter."

Articles appearing in other periodicals include: "The Tragedy of Catherine Thompson [1846]," *Nova Scotia Historical Quarterly*; "The Blast That Rocked Nova Scotia," *Family Practice*; "Dr. Wright's Mechanical Sleigh," *Family Practice*.

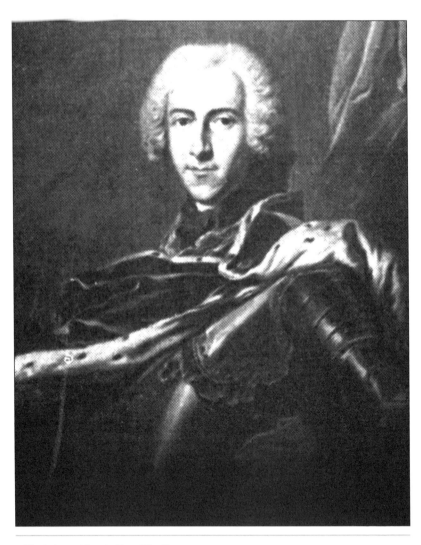

The hale and hearty Duc d'Anville. PUBLIC ARCHIVES OF NOVA SCOTIA

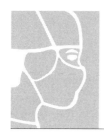

THE DEATH
OF THE FRENCH ARMADA

In May of 1746, the largest military force ever to set sail for the New World was secretly assembled along the French Atlantic coast and departed from Ile Aix. Under the leadership of Admiral Jean-Baptiste Louis Frederic de la Rochefoucauld, the Duc d'Anville, the fleet carried a commission from King Louis XV. They were to avenge the recent stinging defeats of the French at the hands of the English. D'Anville was ordered to "expel the British from Nova Scotia, consign Boston to flames, ravage New England and lay waste to the British West Indies." This was a most ambitious task, but the fleet, consisting of over sixty vessels carrying approximately eleven thousand men, including four battalions of regular French line-infantry, would have been well up to the assignment. Indeed, news of this force created panic in the streets in Boston and New York and sparked mass prayer sessions in colonial churches. But for a series of medical, tactical and climatic misadventures, the Duc d'Anville might even have succeeded in eradicating the English power base in North America.

Things did not go well from the very beginning. Constant delays, possibly caused by the tardiness of shoddy and incompetent contractors, slowed the fleet's departure considerably. Substandard provisions may also have played a role in the subsequent outbreaks of disease on board ship. These delays insured a fatigued and deconditioned crew, even before leaving France. A storm in the Bay of Biscay and adverse winds slowed the trans-Atlantic crossing, the men sickened and began to die as food and drinking water deteriorated. A major storm off Sable Island wrecked and scattered the fleet, and it was a sorry lot of typhus and scurvy-ridden ships that limped into Chebucto Harbour (now Halifax) on September 10, 1746.

And this was only the beginning. Within two weeks of their arrival, the thirty-seven-year-old d'Anville suddenly sickened and died. Sources have listed his death as caused by a variety of conditions including poison, a brain tumour, apoplexy and even the treatment provided by his physicians. A letter written by d'Anville's surgeon and friend Lieutenant Duval, suggests that he fell ill with "a fit of serous apoplexy" (a stroke) sometime during the night of September 24-25 and was found in a vegetative state in his cabin at seven o'clock that morning. Treatment of the Duke proved to be unsuccessful.

On d'Anville's death, Vice Admiral d'Estournelle took command. With 2,500 men dead and much of the fleet and supplies missing, d'Estournelle's situation seemed hopeless. Despondent and discouraged, he repeated over and over, "All is lost; it's impossible." Leaving a meeting with his officers, the depressed vice admiral returned to his cabin. At one point through the night groans were heard coming from his cabin. The officers knocked frantically on the door, then stove it in, to find d'Estournelle lying in a pool of blood, impaled on his own sword.

Third in command, Captain de la Jonquiere, now took command. The sick were brought ashore near Birch Cove in Halifax Harbour's Bedford Basin. Some recovered from scurvy with the arrival of fresh supplies from the Acadians in the Annapolis Valley, but typhus, a louse-borne fever, continued to ravage the men. The feisty Jonquiere determined to at least attempt to take the British fortress of Annapolis Royal on the opposite side of the province to snatch some element of victory. Alas, more storms and English reinforcements resulted in the failure of this plan, and Jonquiere and the remnants of the once grand flotilla limped home to France. Of the approximately eleven thousand men who left France, only a few thousand returned. The prayers of the New Englanders had been answered and there was jubilation in the streets of Boston and New York. Typhus, scurvy, malnutrition, stroke, a brain tumour and depression; all played a role in the failure of this grand scheme of Louis XV.

Dr. Duval had treated the duke with emetics to make him vomit, purges to empty the bowel and blistering which, it was felt then, could suck poisonous substances from the body. Apparently d'Anville initially improved, perhaps due to temporary shrinkage of the tumour brought on by dehydration from his physician's treatment. He briefly regained con-

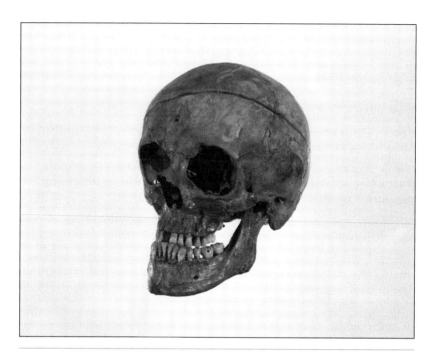

The cranium of the Duc d'Anville, exhumed from beneath the altar at the chapel in Fortress Louisbourg, Cape Breton, showed evidence of a brain tumour that may have caused his fatal stroke. PARKS CANADA / FORTRESS OF LOUISBOURG NATIONAL HISTORIC SITE

sciousness and spoke, but subsequently vomited, aspirated, convulsed and died. Excess fluid in the lungs on autopsy would suggest aspiration as the immediate cause of the duke's death, brought on by loss of consciousness from the tumour-induced stroke.

Dr. Duval performed an autopsy aboard the duke's flagship, *Le Northumberland*, the only autopsy ever to be performed on a royal personage in North America, and he was subsequently buried on Georges Island in Halifax Harbour. Three years later, in 1749, Governor Edward Cornwallis of Halifax gave permission for d'Anville's remains to be "pulled by the heels from his grave" and transferred to Louisbourg. The duke's body was interred with some pomp beneath the altar of the King's Chapel on September 17, 1749. Here the body rested until it was rediscovered in 1932 by workmen excavating the chapel. The identity of the skeleton remained uncertain until the skull was found to house a pig's tooth, one the duke had had implanted two hundred years previously. (This was well known in d'Anville's time and prompted one wag to joke, "He spoke with the tongue of nobility . . . but he laughed with the smile of a pig.")

As often happens after great disasters, the duke's tragic demise piqued the interest of latter day investigators. The skeleton was examined by Dr. J.E. Anderson of McMaster University and was reinterred in Louisbourg in 1964. Here it remained until Halifax neurologist, Dr. Stephen Bedwell, was given permission to examine the remains and make an impression of the skull. Dr. Bedwell also traced a copy of the duke's autopsy report and in combination with his own observations makes a cogent case that the duke may have suffered from a type of brain tumour, called a meningioma. Dr. Duval's autopsy did mention an unusual calcified area (an "ossified scythe") on one fold of the layer of tissue that covers the brain (the dura mater), precisely where one would expect to find a meningioma. Periodic swelling of the tumor would explain d'Anville's headaches and his subsequent collapse with left-sided paralysis from a tumour-associated stroke.

Some tacticians have since pointed out that the fleet would have been far more useful in supporting the Scottish insurrection of Bonnie Prince Charlie. The Highland Scots had invaded England and they might have prevailed if d'Anville had been sent across the Channel with his forces before the decisive Jacobite defeat at Culloden in the month prior to his departure.

The most tangible result of d'Anville's expedition was to prompt the British government to found the city of Halifax at Chebucto in 1749. The strong garrison here anchored the English presence, and likely prevented Nova Scotia from joining the other American Colonies when they successfully rebelled during the Revolutionary War.

Just think: but for d'Anville, we could all be saluting the Stars and Stripes right now!

George Burden

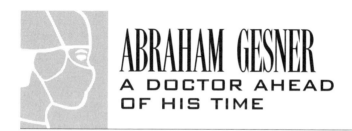

ABRAHAM GESNER

A DOCTOR AHEAD OF HIS TIME

He did more to save the great whales than probably any other individual in history. He was a civil rights activist one hundred years before it became fashionable. He laid the foundations for the modern petrochemical industry, yet showed a keen insight into waste control and pollution prevention. Abraham Gesner was by training a physician, a GP (a general practitioner, now usually called a Family Physician) who practiced in the little town of Parrsboro in Nova Scotia almost two centuries ago. Like many talented Canadians, his story is little known to most people.

Gesner was born into genteel poverty on May 2, 1797, to Henry and Sarah Gesner. Growing up on a farm in Cornwallis, Kings County, Nova Scotia, young Abraham's education was limited, due to his family's impoverished state. By age twenty-four, the young man's situation was desperate. Without education and nearly bankrupt, he was in love with Harriet Webster, the daughter of a prosperous local physician, Dr. Isaac Webster. The young couple married, and Harriet's father agreed to bail the young man out of debt, but only if Abraham would agree to go to England to study medicine. While medicine did not especially interest Gesner, he had no other choice and soon found himself in London studying at Guy's and St. Bartholemew's hospitals. His great intellectual loves were chemistry and geology, and in addition to his medical studies, Gesner attended lectures on these subjects. At age thirty he returned home to set up practice in Parrsboro.

This small village, located on the Bay of Fundy, was a geological treasure trove, and Gesner interspersed his medical practice with collecting expeditions and surveys of the coal- and fossil-rich cliffs of his new home.

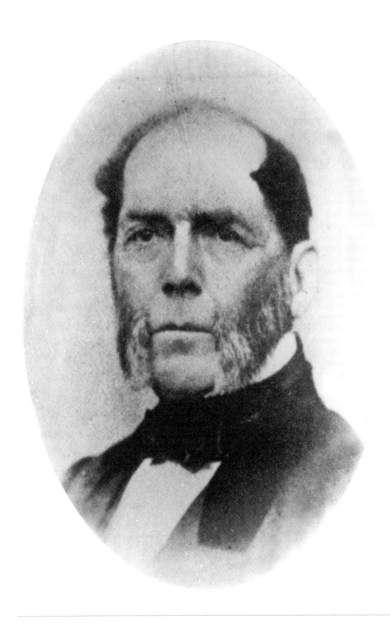

Dr. Abraham Gesner, the founder of the modern petrochemical industry.

During his wanderings, he made many friends among the Mi'kmaq in the province, and later proved to be a strong advocate for this people. Gesner was a great proponent of smallpox immunization among European and native peoples alike. He also proved to be a vocal critic of the dumping of fish offal and waste into the Bay of Fundy and later developed a technique for recycling this waste as fertilizer. In addition to ministering to local health needs, he would often liven up the isolated cabins of his clientele with the sound of his flute.

Eventually Gesner gave up his medical practice in Parrsboro, and such was his prestige in geology that in 1838 the government of New Brunswick hired him to do a geological survey of the province. By then he was acknowledged to be the greatest authority on this subject in Maritime Canada. The position also offered financial security to Gesner whose burgeoning offspring placed a large economic demand on the family.

While in New Brunswick, he set the groundwork for Canada's first museum, the Saint John Museum, with the collection he began under the auspices of the Mechanics' Institute. Gesner's son was later to relate how all winter long his father's Mi'kmaq guides lived and laboured in the attic of the family home, mounting specimens for the museum. In 1842 Gesner was honoured by Sir Charles Lyell, the great English geologist, with a request to guide him on his explorations of the Maritimes.

His years in New Brunswick were marred by a vicious and libelous letter campaign spearheaded by a jealous physician colleague, Dr. James Robb. In 1843 Gesner decided to leave the province and return to Cornwallis, Nova Scotia. This move was no doubt fueled by his increasingly vociferous critics and by his father's increasing age and inability to manage the family farm on his own.

Although setting early productivity records in Cornwallis by using a new fertilizer he developed from apple-processing waste, the disastrous harvest of 1848 finally forced him to sell the property. Nevertheless, Gesner's prospects looked good, for while living in New Brunswick he had developed a process for extracting a high-quality illuminating gas, as well as an oil he called "kerosene," from Albertite ore. This mineral, similar to asphalt or bitumen, was named for its place of discovery, Albert County, New Brunswick.

The name kerosene derived from the Greek *keros* and *elaion*, meaning respectively "wax" and "oil." Kerosene proved to be an excellent and cheap alternative to whale oil for lighting purposes. Gesner also invented a type of lantern suitable for burning his new discovery. Unintentionally, he had knocked the bottom out of the whale oil market and significantly reduced the slaughter of cetaceans. Many feel that the great whales would already be extinct but for his timely discovery.

In 1846, he did a geological survey of Prince Edward Island and also had great success lecturing on his findings. Gesner was a forceful and charismatic speaker, and audiences always flocked to hear him. Not forgetting medicine entirely, Gesner also advocated that a summer cholera outbreak in Charlottetown could be stemmed by piping a clean source of fresh water from nearby Grey's Spring.

Moving back to Nova Scotia, Gesner became Commissioner of Indian Affairs. Appalled at the state of the Mi'kmaq nation, he organized a protest at the Nova Scotia legislature in 1849. Accompanied by ten Mi'kmaq chiefs in full regalia, he was greeted cordially by Lt. Governor Sir John Harvey. Little was accomplished by this rally except to damage Gesner's reputation further in the eyes of the reactionary powers in Halifax.

Unfortunately, Gesner was never able to obtain much financial benefit from his discoveries, due to opposition from well-financed monopolies such as Nova Scotia's General Mining Association (GMA). Several disastrous and expensive lawsuits were all decided against him, and he found himself in worse financial straits than ever. This was in spite of the fact that the city of Washington D.C. had adopted his Albertite gas to light the American capital. Gesner's old nemesis, Dr. Robb, actually did an about face and supported his former rival's claims, but to no avail. Ten years after Gesner's proposal to gaslight the city of Saint John was turned down, the city hired an American company to accomplish that task.

In the face of these disappointments, Gesner decided to move to New York. The Americans had a greater appreciation for his talents than had his fellow Maritimers, and he was promptly snapped up by the newly formed Asphalt Mining and Kerosene Gas Company. Here he continued to expand on his work with kerosene, pioneering the modern petrochemical industry.

Living in Brooklyn, Gesner's son later related how at church picnics his kindhearted father would pass barrels of food across the fence to starving urchins. In 1859, Dr. Gesner, at age sixty-two, lost his job with the Kerosene Gas Company due to a changeover in production techniques. He practiced medicine for a while in New York, then returned to Nova Scotia, working for a while on a fertilizer called "Artificial Guano," and later tried his hand at gold prospecting. Still destitute, he applied to Dalhousie University in Halifax for a professorship of Chemistry and Natural History. Unfortunately, on the board of the college was one of the principals of the Halifax Gas Company, another company with which Gesner had feuded in the course of asserting his claims. His application was rejected and a Dr. Lawson from Toronto was offered the post.

Gesner died in April 1864. No mention was made in his obituary of the doctor's many accomplishments, and he was buried in an unmarked grave in the Camp Hill Cemetery in Halifax. In 1933, Imperial Oil finally erected a monument commemorating this great Canadian, the neglected founder of the petroleum refining industry, a pioneering environmentalist and the saviour of the great whales.

George Burden

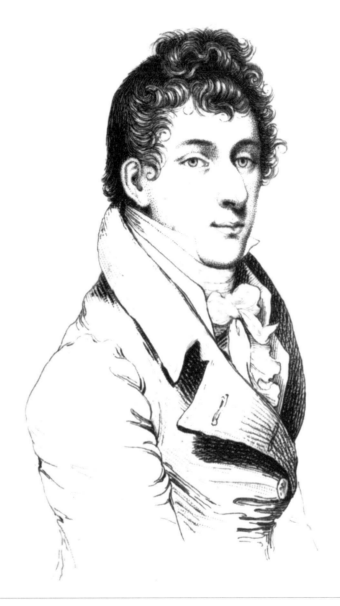

Handsome, intelligent and refined, sociopath Henry Moon conned and cheated his way across North America. NEW BRUNSWICK MUSEUM

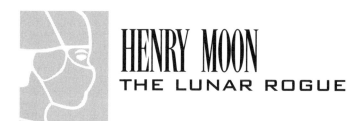

HENRY MOON
THE LUNAR ROGUE

Mr. Henry Moon spoke and carried himself like an English gentleman. He was handsome, dressed elegantly and could be exceedingly charming. He spoke French fluently, played the violin and had the manual dexterity to craft almost anything with very little in the way of raw materials. Henry could preach better than most ministers and had many verses of the Old and New Testaments committed to memory. He was also a cunning and masterful liar and a talented thief who could pick locks and enter and leave homes at night with great facility. Though endowed with a genius that would have allowed him to earn a good living honestly, Mr. Moon delighted in duping and conning his fellow man, at times in wickedly humorous ways.

Little is known of Moon prior to his appearance in the community of Rawdon, Nova Scotia, in 1812. He introduced himself as an Englishman, a tailor by trade, and assumed the alias of Henry More Smith. He sought employment with wealthy sawmill-owner John Bond and for about a year passed for an honest, hard-working employee. His fellow employees distrusted him, however, and there was a rumour that he was "in league with the devil." In a folk tale still extant in Rawdon, Moon was asked to cut up a pile of wood at the lumber camp one evening. He told his fellows that "the Black Man" (i.e. Satan) would do it for him and retired to bed. The next morning the wood was cut, and the smell of brimstone was in the air. No doubt Moon had sneaked out and cut the wood in the dark of the night, leaving a pinch of sulphur on the dying campfire, thus fooling his gullible brethren. With stories like these, it is no wonder Bond refused Henry's request for his daughter Elizabeth's hand. This, however, did not deter the couple, who eloped in March 1813.

Henry set up business as a tailor and peddler, travelling to Halifax to ply his trade each afternoon and returning the next morning. People noticed that these were not normal business hours, and when the true owner recognized a coat Henry had "tailored" for a customer, it became evident he had been spending his nights cleverly burgling the citizenry of Halifax. He set off, abandoning his wife, and fled to New Brunswick.

Moon robbed and conned his way through the countryside, eventually making the error of stealing the favourite bay mare of Farmer Knox. He was captured and later claimed that Farmer Knox had given him a few "knocks" on his way to the Kingston Jail where he came into the custody of Sheriff Walter Bates, who has written a book about his experiences with Henry Moon. The handsome and charming prisoner elicited a lot of sympathy from the locals. Protesting his innocence, he began to complain of increasing pain in his chest, pointing to an ugly bruise where he alleged that Knox had pistol-whipped him. The prisoner's condition deteriorated to the point where it was felt he had little time to live and physician Adino Paddock, Jr. was summoned. With his patient febrile and vomiting blood the doctor felt little could be done to help him. Townsfolk brought the prisoner gifts of cordials and a down comforter to lie on in his last hours. Henry gasped that he would not survive the night and asked one of the assistant jailers to bring him a hot brick to warm his dying body. The jailer hastened to do so, leaving the door open, and upon his return he found Moon gone. Later a passerby described what he thought was the ghost of Henry hurrying across a field.

Inexplicably, rather than making his escape to nearby American territory, Moon remained in the vicinity continuing to rob and con the locals out of substantial amounts of goods and money. He even had the audacity to rob the home of the Attorney General by venturing into his porch while he was having a party and making off with the guests' hats and coats. However, when he impulsively invited himself to breakfast at a local farm and in a conversational manner admitted he was the one the authorities were looking for, he was arrested again.

Back in Kingston, Moon's jailers were determined that he would not escape a second time and placed him in chains. The prisoner repeatedly tore off or sawed through his chains with small homemade implements. Sheriff Bates describes how Moon twisted a one-and-a-half-inch-wide

THE MYSTERIOUS STRANGER;

—— OR ——

MEMOIRS OF THE NOTED

HENRY MORE SMITH,

·——— CONTAINING ———·

A correct account of his extraordinary conduct during the
thirteen months of his confinement in the Jail of King's
County, Province of New Brunswick, where he
was convicted of Horse Stealing, and
under sentence of death.

—— ALSO ——

A Sketch of his Life and Character

From his first appearance at Windsor, in Nova Scotia, in the
year 1812, to the time of his apprehension and confinement.

TO WHICH IS ADDED

A HISTORY OF HIS CAREER

EMBRACING AN ACCOUNT OF HIS

IMPRISONMENTS AND ESCAPES,

Selected from the most authentic sources, both public and private.

BY WALTER BATES, Esquire.

SAINT JOHN, N. B.:
PRINTED BY GEO. W. DAY, CORNER PRINCE WM. AND PRINCESS STS.
1887.

The title page of Walter Bates's much reprinted biography of the notorious Henry
Moon, alias Henry More Smith. GEORGE BURDEN

steel collar as if it were made of leather. Heavier and heavier chains were employed until the prisoner had almost fifty pounds of metal hanging from his body, yet he still managed to greet his jailer in the morning with scarcely a link intact.

Still unable to effect an escape, Moon began to act in a quite insane manner. He screamed and yelled all night, showing no recognition of anyone. This went on for months, and, despite an admirable performance at his trial, Henry Moon was informed that he was going to be sentenced to hang for horse thievery.

Henry then attempted to elicit sympathy from the prison guards. Incredibly, he was able to fashion lifelike mannequins of his wife praying over him, so realistic that viewers were moved to pity. Subsequently he fashioned a "family" of tiny puppets: men, women, children and infants, and tiny musicians who would beat a drum or tambourine. All were remarkably lifelike. He did this in the dark, chained, and using only straw, clothing ripped from his body, soot and his own blood for colouring. People came from all over and paid money to see Moon's exhibitions at which he would play the fiddle accompanied by his puppet percussionists and dancers. Dr. Couglen, an Irish military surgeon, commented that he had not seen anything so remarkable in his travels around the world.

Henry's ploy worked. He predicted to his jailer that he would receive a pardon, and that is exactly what happened. He was released and took passage on a boat to Nova Scotia, where he again stole enough to finance passage to the United States. Ironically, he abandoned his little family of puppets, which could have earned him a good deal of honest money. Continuing his trade of larceny, Moon travelled through the eastern United States under various aliases and served several prison terms. For a while he was a successful evangelist in the southern states. Years later, Moon travelled to Upper Canada and visited Augustus Bates, the brother of his former jailer. Again exhibiting his perverse sense of humour, Moon passed himself off as a good friend of the High Sheriff. He set up in town and took deposits on a shipment of non-existent goods he claimed to have smuggled in duty-free from the United States. The last we hear of Moon is about 1835 when a man fitting his description was incarcerated in the Toronto Gaol. Sheriff Bates was not well enough to travel to Upper

Canada to verify the prisoner's identity, and thus end the chronicles of Mr. Henry Moon.

In short, Moon was a sociopath, a man with no conscience. His behaviour, as chronicled by Walter Bates, may be the first definitive case history of this disorder in Canada. The good sheriff meticulously followed Moon's antics from 1812 to 1835 in his book, *The Mysterious Stranger*. The information Sheriff Bates provides clearly shows that Mr. Moon meets the criteria of an Antisocial Personality Disorder as laid out in the *Diagnostic and Statistical Manual*, the bible of the psychiatric profession today. Requiring only three or more of seven criteria to make a diagnosis, Henry appears to satisfy five of them: "(1) failure to conform to social norms with respect to lawful behaviors . . . (2) deceitfulness . . . repeated lying . . . conning others (3) impulsivity and failing to plan ahead (4) consistent irresponsibility . . . failure to sustain consistent work behavior and (5) lack of remorse" (over his deeds).

Though known to be irritable and to utter threats, Henry departs from the behaviour of many sociopaths in that he never physically harmed anyone or attempted violence towards another human being. This, coupled with his charm and roguish sense of humour, has endeared Moon to many throughout the last two centuries.

George Burden

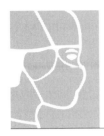

CATHERINE ANN THOMPSON
THE SILENCED WITNESS

It began with a death. In this case, it was the death of a middle-aged woman who had been, according to her relatives, mentally ill for many years.

The Reverend Father James Kennedy officiated at her funeral on September 22, 1846. He knew very little about the deceased except that she was the aunt of Mary Thompson, wife of Colonel George Forbes Thompson, a retired English army officer. It was a depressing, rainy day, and the salt-laced wind off Halifax harbour mounded soggy remnants of leaves around the open grave. As the priest murmured the last words of prayer, he turned to the two mourners who stood with him in the small cemetery. In a gesture of sympathy, he placed a comforting hand on the shoulder of the dead woman's niece.

What Father Kennedy didn't know was the fact that the couple had good reason to be greatly relieved by the woman's death. Any sense of relief, however, must have been quickly dispelled when, soon after the funeral, a coroner's inquest opened in Dartmouth. Its role was to investigate allegations that Mary had murdered her aunt.

To set the stage for the inquest, it is important to introduce the main characters in the plot. First, the Colonel, George Forbes Thompson. He had come to Nova Scotia in 1845 intending to settle in Aylesford, King's County, but instead decided to purchase a large estate at Dartmouth's Lake Loon. The Colonel's charm and affluence impressed the local gentry. Then there is Mary, his beautiful, red-haired companion, who did not enjoy a similar review. Much younger than Thompson, she was not a lady of high breeding, as her habit of screaming and cursing made clear. Visitors to the Thompson's elaborate home were often left with the feeling that it would be difficult to find two people less suited to each other.

Added to the gossip that began to circulate about the couple was the rumour that Mary's unmarried aunt was living in appalling conditions. Servants reported that the pathetic woman was kept locked up in a small, closet-like, poorly heated room, and no one was allowed near her unless accompanied by one of the Thompsons. Even at a time when a terrible stigma was attached to insanity, the servants were shocked by the meagre diet they were ordered to prepare for this seemingly harmless woman.

One day, while the Thompsons were away visiting Halifax, a group of small children happened to wander into their garden. Playing near the house, they were suddenly frightened by a shrill voice calling out to them. Looking up they saw a thin, unkempt woman standing at a second floor window. Speaking with a strange accent, she repeated the same two sentences. "I am the real Mrs. Thompson. Mary is an impostor!" The woman also complained about Mary who, she claimed, was masquerading as the Colonel's wife, and she insisted that this wicked person was treating her cruelly.

This story, told by the children, prompted more speculation about the Thompsons. After all, people asked, why was Mary's harmless aunt kept a prisoner in their home? And what about her declaration that she was "the real Mrs. Thompson?" Could this possibly be true? But before anyone could actively investigate the bizarre circumstances of the mystery woman, Colonel Thompson made a significant announcement. He told his friends and neighbours that Mary's very frail aunt had passed away. According to him, she died peacefully in his arms during the early evening hours of September 20, 1846. (It was later learned that he had not been present when the woman passed away.)

Then Thompson did something that surprised many people. Although both he and Mary attended an Anglican Church, he now made arrangements for the dead woman to be buried in a Roman Catholic cemetery. Catholics who heard of his decision began to raise questions about the circumstances of the woman's death and were distressed to learn that the Thompsons had not arranged for their relative to receive the last rites, a sacred ritual for all dying Catholics.

Local authorities soon found themselves besieged by people who demanded that they investigate the woman's death. On September 29, 1846, their pleas were acknowledged, and a coroner's inquest began at Hoyne's Hotel, on Queen Street in Dartmouth. Fortunately, someone had learned that some of the army officers who had once served with Thompson were now located in Halifax. These men would certainly know whether the dead woman had been telling the truth about being the Colonel's wife. With this intriguing possibility in mind, the body was exhumed. Two local doctors performed an autopsy and reported their findings at a packed hearing. They testified that there was no evidence the woman had met a violent death. They did, however, disclose that they had seldom seen such a shocking case of malnutrition and that there was little doubt the deceased woman had suffered from an advanced case of tuberculosis.

Next, two army officers took the stand. Both stated that they had known Thompson's wife during the years when the Colonel, like themselves, had been stationed in Barbados. They identified the emaciated body as being that of their old friend, Catherine Thompson. The officers also testified that this gaunt corpse was only a shadow of the attractive woman who had lived with the Colonel during his time in the West Indies. Several days of confused and varied testimony by the Thompsons' servants did little to help the jury come to a decision. Mary, the mistress of the house, had never been known to pamper her staff and more than one former housemaid was delighted to publicly disclose some of the distasteful aspects of her employer's obnoxious personality.

Today, more than a hundred and fifty years later, the Public Archives of Nova Scotia retain the coroner's report of that hearing. For a researcher, it presents another mysterious component of this fascinating story. The faded and dog-eared document states that the woman whose death was attributed to "lack of care," was indeed Catherine Ann Thompson. But, strangely, this name has been scratched out and, in the space above it is written: "a woman whose name is to the jurors unknown," and the verdict issued on October 6, 1846, states that "the jurors had strong reason to believe she was the wife of Colonel Thompson, but they were unable to account for her death."

Unfortunately, it is impossible to completely decipher the faded writing on the inquest's documents. This means that it would be a quite a challenge to determine on what basis the jury finally concluded that George Thompson and Mary should be found innocent of all charges. In the eyes of the public, the couple were criminals who had managed to avoid the justice they deserved. People felt that there were far too many questions left unanswered. For example, why had Thompson tried to prevent exhumation of the body? Why had he refused to allow any of his old army friends to visit his Dartmouth home? And how did he explain the frequent arguments he had with Mary? Servants insisted that they heard Mary demanding that he marry her.

The army officers had testified that Catherine Ann Thompson was of Spanish origin. Could this explain why some of the Thompsons' servants had mentioned that the poor woman had spoken with "a foreign accent" and that she had frequently asked for wine? Colonel Thompson insisted that his wife's "aunt" had never married, yet the doctors who examined the body were convinced that she had given birth to several children. Perhaps the most important flaw in the Colonel's testimony was his statement that his first wife had died in 1835. The army officers who knew him were baffled by this declaration since they were adamant that they had met Catherine several years after this date.

Although Thompson and Mary continued to insist they had done nothing wrong, the public at large remained convinced that the woman buried in the Roman Catholic cemetery was George Thompson's legal wife. They also believed the Thompsons were responsible for her death.

A few months later the Colonel sold his home and, with Mary, returned to England. Their departure did not end speculations about the case. Local writers, unable to rest until the truth was revealed, began to construct the true story of the dead woman who was left behind in a Dartmouth cemetery. Like amateur detectives, they searched for clues that would help them recapture some sense of Catherine Thompson's lost identity.

Catherine Ann Thompson, it is alleged, was once described as being one of the most beautiful girls on the island of Gibraltar. The daughter of a wealthy Spanish merchant and his Scottish wife, she could have had her pick of any of the eligible officers stationed at the Spanish or English garrison. Sadly, she made the mistake of falling in love with George Thompson, a young, arrogant English ensign.

Thompson was addicted to gambling, and Catherine's sizeable dowry was impressive enough to convince him to forsake his single life. But being a bit of a scallywag, once her dowry was spent, he neglected his wife and took no interest in the children born to them. Several years after their wedding, Thompson's regiment was posted to Barbados. The posting came at a tumultuous time; the family arrived on the island during a period of widespread unrest. One night, while Thompson was away at his garrison, a new riot broke out. Hundreds of Barbadians rushed into the English section of Bridgetown. Soon houses were burning and many men, women and children became victims of mob mentality. One of the homes the rioters invaded was the Thompson family residence.

Terrified by the intrusion, Catherine had managed to hide two of her children in closets, but before she could find a hiding place for herself and her baby son, the angry mob was rushing up the stairs to the second floor. Kicking down a door, they burst into the bedroom where she was cowering. The invaders brutally tore her infant from her arms, and, as she watched in horror, they threw the child out of a window to the pavement below. When Thompson returned home, he found his wife murmuring incoherently, rocking the dead baby in her arms. The Thompsons returned to England a shattered family. Catherine was placed in a mental institution and their children sent to private schools.

The story might well have ended here except for the fact that George Thompson's regiment was later sent to Ceylon where he met a young Irish woman named Mary Taylor. The widow of a sergeant who had served in Thompson's regiment, she was only too eager to become the well-to-do colonel's housekeeper. She soon developed an intimate relationship with him. Some writers report that while the couple lived together in Ceylon, she gave birth to a child. It is known that Mary gave birth to a son while she was living in Nova Scotia.

The birth of her first child was of momentous significance to Mary. Realizing her children would have no legal claims to their father's estate as long as Catherine was alive, she decided that she must find a way to marry George Thompson. The opportunity she was looking for came when Thompson retired from the army and was considering moving to Nova Scotia. Mary eagerly endorsed the idea. She probably suggested they take Catherine along with the excuse that, if Mary cared for her, Thompson would be able to save a great deal of money. To avoid gossip, she insisted they tell people that Catherine was her aunt.

Why did Thompson agree to her plan? Probably because he knew there was no way he could legally rid himself of Catherine, and he was tired of Mary's demands that he "do right by her." In Nova Scotia, he did nothing to prevent Catherine's death and allowed Mary to neglect and mistreat his wife. Was Catherine murdered? It seems the nineteenth-century jury was not convinced.

Sadly, even the people who had once deplored her unnecessary death soon forgot Catherine. Ironically, across the ocean, a first cousin was enjoying the splendour of a royal court. She became the Empress Eugenie, wife of Napoleon III, and earned a permanent place in history. Catherine's fate could not have been more different. It was her destiny to witness the murder of a baby, to lose her remaining children and to suffer cruel neglect at the hands of two despicable people.

Today, all that is known about Catherine's final resting place is that her mortal remains lie in an unmarked grave somewhere in a small Dartmouth cemetery far away from her Spanish homeland and from those who once truly loved her.

Dorothy Grant

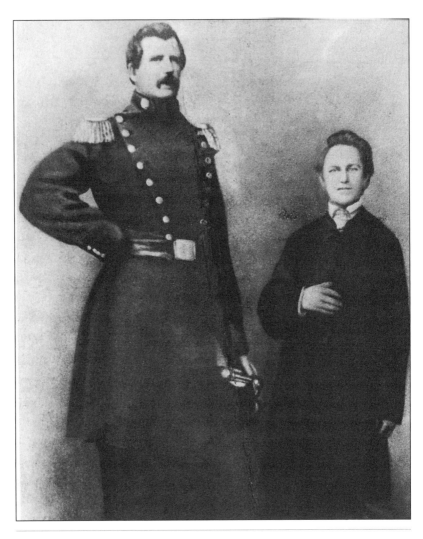

The elegantly attired Cape Breton giant towers over a companion in this formal portrait. PUBLIC ARCHIVES OF NOVA SCOTIA

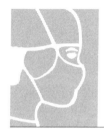

ANGUS McASKILL
A GIANT AMONG MEN

It might be something in the salt air of the province, or perhaps it is the vast amount of seafood that Bluenosers consume. Whatever the reason, nineteenth-century Nova Scotia produced some of the biggest human beings ever to live. One of these was Angus McAskill. Born in the Hebrides off the west coast of Scotland, Angus was a smallish child when his family emigrated to Englishtown on Cape Breton Island. One of thirteen children of Norman and Christina McAskill, he was unremarkable until the age of twelve when something strange happened. Young Angus began to tower over his classmates. Larger kids used to thrash him regularly in schoolyard wrestling matches. Now they started to run the other way, fast, when they saw Angus coming. He quickly gained the nickname of *gille mhor* or "big boy" in the Gaelic widely spoken in Cape Breton.

Soon Norman McAskill had to begin major renovations to his home, raising the ceilings and constructing a specially reinforced eight-foot-long bed for his young son. Angus was a gentle, patient and religious young man who usually took his share of teasing with great forbearance. One lapse is recorded, however. When he was thirteen and working as a cabin boy, he attended a dance in North Sydney. Following the nautical custom of the day, Angus was barefoot and simply chose to sit on the sidelines and enjoy the dancers and music. One prankster, however, found great amusement in repeatedly stepping on Angus's unshod toes. After the third time, Angus could take no more. He stood up and punched his tormentor in the face, sending him flying to the centre of the room, out cold. Deeply sorry afterwards, Angus successfully prayed for his victim's recovery.

Hard work on his father's farm ensured that Angus grew not only in height but in strength as well. On one occasion, a neighbour bet Norman

McAskill ten dollars he couldn't plow one of his fields by sundown. The bet looked like a certain loss when one of the horses went lame until Angus harnessed himself cheek by jowl with the remaining horse and started pulling. Father and son would likely have won the bet, too, except that Christina McAskill felt that Angus looked too undignified in the traces. Rushing from the farmhouse, her skirts in a flurry, she made him stop.

On another occasion, Norman McAskill and two other men had tried repeatedly, without success, to lift an especially heavy log onto a rack for sawing. They left in disgust, but on their return they discovered the log in its place. Young Angus claimed to have completed the task single-handedly. At first the men refused to believe him, but the lad tossed the log back into the pit, then returned it to the rack as they watched incredulously.

By the time he was in his early twenties, Angus weighed nearly five hundred pounds, was seven feet nine inches tall, and wore size fourteen-and-a-half shoes. His fame began to spread, and he became a target for bullies trying to make a name fighting the lad. Being passive and gentle by nature, he generally refused, often rousing the ire of his antagonists. A three-hundred-pound American fishing captain became so rude and insistent that Angus finally picked him up and tossed him over a ten-foot haystack.

As more and more people heard about Angus, he received offers to go on tour to other parts of Canada and to the United States. On one occasion, bandits attempted to rob the train in which the giant was travelling. McAskill stood up to his full seven feet nine inches, glared at the bandits and flexed his muscles, sending the malefactors racing from the train. The giant frequently toured with the famous midget, Colonel Tom Thumb. Crowds loved it when Angus displayed his diminutive partner standing in the palm of his hand.

Angus later visited England and was presented to Queen Victoria at Windsor Castle. The ruler of the world's largest empire chatted amiably with perhaps the largest of her subjects, and both were charmed. Victoria left Angus with gifts and her compliments.

While he was touring in the United States, several sailors challenged McAskill to lift an anchor that weighed in excess of two thousand pounds. He successfully accomplished the task, even taking the heavy object for a short walk around the dock. But somehow his load slipped as he was setting it down, and he fell, taking the full impact of the anchor onto his body. Some say he was never the same after this and that the injury may have hastened his demise. In any event, this was Angus's last tour. In the early 1850s he retired home to Englishtown, now affluent from his earnings abroad, and opened a grocery and dry goods store. A kind-hearted and charitable man, he never let the needy leave his store empty-handed. Later, McAskill purchased a gristmill, ensuring its profitability by pushing the millstones himself when water levels were too low.

As time went on, Angus McAskill's health began to fail. On August 1, 1863, he developed a sudden illness, and seven days later the largest and perhaps strongest citizen of British North America was dead at the age of thirty-four. His physician diagnosed "brain fever" as the cause of death. A contemporary medical reference (*Buchan's Domestic Medicine*) describes this as a febrile illness characterized by "pain of the head, redness of the eyes, a violent flushing of the face . . ., blood from the nose, singing of the ears and extreme sensibility of the nervous system." The volume states that brain fever or "phrenitis" often followed other infections, and this ailment likely represents meningitis in modern diagnostic terms.

It seems probable that Angus McAskill suffered from hyperpituitarism, with excessive secretion of growth hormone as the cause of his great stature. It is documented that even in adulthood, his hands and feet continued to grow, so we know he suffered from acromegaly, the adult manifestation of elevated growth hormone. His life expectancy, especially in the nineteenth century, would have been limited due to this ailment. People suffering from hyperpituitarism often develop congestive heart failure, hypertension and diabetes. General debility from one or more of these complications would have made McAskill even more prone to develop an infectious illness such as meningitis.

It took six hours and the labour of two carpenters to build Angus's huge coffin. Three men floated the coffin to its final destination, a churchyard overlooking the scenic waters of Englishtown's St. Ann's Bay. A large group of friends and neighbours gathered for the final sendoff of their huge, gentle and well-loved giant.

George Burden

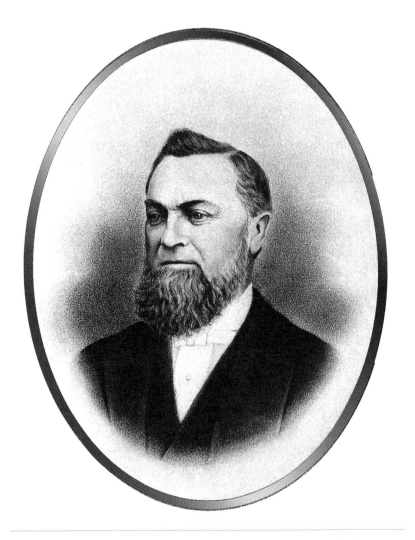

The Reverend John Cameron, a fiery preacher, proved equally adept at healing the souls and the disease-wracked bodies of his parishioners. BRIDGETOWN AND AREA HERITAGE SOCIETY

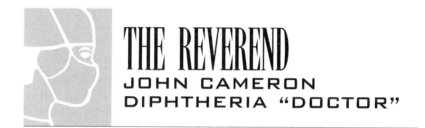

THE REVEREND
JOHN CAMERON
DIPHTHERIA "DOCTOR"

The village of Elmsdale, Nova Scotia, where I practice, has European roots going back to 1785. That is when the first land grants were made to settlers at the V-shaped confluence of the Shubenacadie and Nine Mile rivers, where the village is nestled. For centuries prior to this, the area was a meeting place for the Mi'kmaq people who used the lakes and rivers of our province as a natural highway. After the Napoleonic Wars, settlers appeared in the region in greater numbers, but the area contained only a few scattered farmsteads with no focal point until three fateful events occurred: the construction of a canal system, the building of a railroad and, not least, the appearance on the scene of a fiery and determined preacher, the Reverend John Cameron.

On September 17, 1844, just four days shy of his twenty-seventh birthday, John Cameron was inducted at the one poor church in the area. He was the only clergyman for many miles around, and had inherited a parish with much lawlessness. The hard-drinking and profane denizens of the local gold mines and lumber camps patronized the saloons and licensed boarding houses in the community, making the streets unpleasant and sometimes unsafe for more law-abiding residents. In his first year, Reverend Cameron covered thirty-five hundred miles of trails on horseback, spreading the gospel to often-isolated households. Suffering ill health, he spent the winter of 1845 to1846 in Philadelphia. Realizing that there was very little available in the way of medical care in his home con-stituency, Cameron supplemented his knowledge of the Lord by attending medical lectures at Philadelphia medical colleges, obtaining information which was to prove invaluable in his later ministrations.

By 1858, the good reverend had whipped the lawless township into a

God-fearing community. Even the miners knew better than to incur the wrath of Cameron and were behaving themselves. Not so *Corynebacterium diphtheriae*, the causative agent for diphtheria, which was ravaging the province. Records show that in the nearby community of Shubenacadie, a hundred and fifty people were infected and eighty died from the disease. The illness caused a greyish-white membrane to form in the throat of its victims, and in addition to blocking the upper airways, this bacterial growth produced toxins or poisons which spread through the blood stream to other parts of the body. The membrane made breathing difficult, if not impossible, and the toxin affected the heart and nerves, causing inflammation and damage to these organs. At the time, the only known treatment was the application of caustic soda to the infected tissues of the throat, which presumably shrank the thick membrane and kept it from obstructing the airway. (It's ironic that I have patients now who absolutely refuse immunization against an agent which was killing their great-grandparents in such large numbers.)

Cameron was not one to let his parishioners die off while he did nothing. He had no caustic soda on hand, so he fired off a note by messenger to the doctor in Shubenacadie, asking for the loan of some caustic soda until he could order his own supply from Halifax. Not only did the local physician refuse to supply the material, but he also threatened legal action if Cameron treated anyone. (I would like to think this was done out of concern for untrained personnel managing the deadly ailment and not from fear of competition and financial loss.) Undeterred, Cameron undertook the arduous horseback ride to Halifax. There, his friend Dr. Parker trusted the cleric's medical abilities more than did his colleague in Shubenacadie and happily provided the reverend with the needed caustic soda. For the next two months John Cameron seldom got any rest, working night and day to save, not the souls, but the lives of his flock. The church elders reportedly said, "Forget the sermons; they can wait. Look after the sick." Implementing what he had learned in Philadelphia about the treatment of disease, in conjunction with some new information on the importance of sanitation, Cameron attended nearly two hundred people in his district, and it was said that not one of them died. After the epidemic settled, his grateful parishioners voted him ten pounds cash and a fine horse, a very handsome gift indeed for those times.

We do not know whether Reverend Cameron was called on to provide medical care on such a large scale again. We can presume that in the absence of a doctor he continued — when required — to tend to the physical needs of his flock. He looked after the spiritual needs of his little community in Elmsdale and the surrounding area until 1879. Then he moved to Bridgetown, Nova Scotia, where he continued to work until his death in 1907 at the age of ninety and in the sixty-third year of his ministry. A plaque can still be seen in Elmsdale's hundred-and-fifty-year-old Presbyterian church, commemorating Cameron's thirty-three years of service there. He chose to be buried in Elmsdale's little community cemetery, where a simple headstone marks the final resting place of this remarkable man, a cleric by profession and a physician by necessity.

George Burden

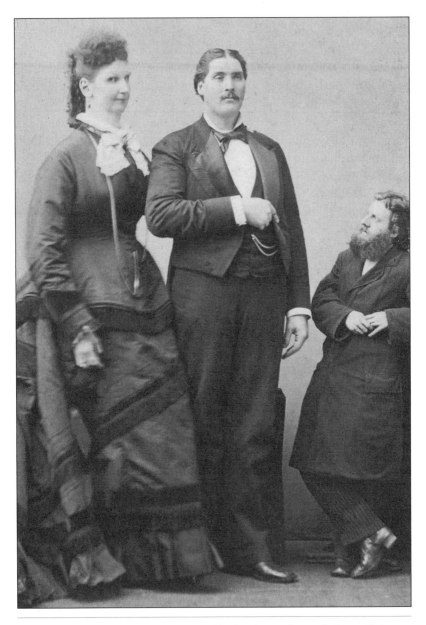

The giantess Anna Swan with her beloved husband, Captain Martin Bates. Their great stature brought them triumph, tragedy and a place in the *Guinness Book of World Records*. DALE SWAN / PUBLIC ARCHIVES OF NOVA SCOTIA

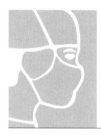

ANNA SWAN
THE GENTLE GIANTESS

This is a tale of love and passion and tragedy, and its protagonist was almost eight feet tall.

I refer to the life of Anna Swan, the Canadian giantess who astounded the world in the mid-nineteenth century. Anna was fated to be wooed away to New York City by P.T. Barnum and to be feted by Queen Victoria and the monarchs of Europe, but her life began simply with her birth in the tiny village of Millbrook, Nova Scotia. The third of twelve children, she was born on August 6, 1846, and her parents knew something was a bit odd when their new baby girl weighed in a thirteen pounds. By age four, Anna was almost fifty inches high, and by age seven she had outgrown her mother. Soon after, she towered over her five-foot-six-inch father, and at seventeen she measured seven foot eleven and a half inches and weighed over four hundred pounds. Her shoes, clothing and bed had to be custom-made. Ordinary chairs would not hold her, so she simply sat on the kitchen floor at mealtime.

Anna was a bright student, though special measures had to be taken in the school to accommodate her gargantuan dimensions. She later attended the Normal School in Truro, with aspirations of becoming a teacher. Though massive in size, her gentle nature attracted children to her. By 1862, however, the famous impresario, Phineas T. Barnum, had succeeded in luring Anna to New York to become a part of his American Museum. Mr. and Mrs. Swan, determined to see their daughter treated with proper decorum and respect, accompanied her to New York. Anna's regimen at the museum included tutoring and music lessons, and she entertained her visitors by giving lectures, acting in plays and performing on the piano.

She was well paid by the day's standard, twenty-three dollars per week, in gold coinage.

Unfortunately, the museum burned down in 1865, costing Anna her money and belongings and almost taking her life. As she was unable to descend flame-weakened stairs, rescuers broke a hole in the wall of the building and lowered the giantess to the ground with a derrick. Anna then returned to Nova Scotia, but later she rejoined Barnum in a rebuilt American Museum. This museum also was destroyed by fire in 1868, and the discouraged Barnum went into semi-retirement.

Undeterred, Anna joined a group of entertainers who were touring the United States, and while attending a party in New Jersey, she met Captain Martin Van Buren Bates, the seven-foot-nine-inch "Kentucky Giant." Bates had been a Confederate officer during the United States Civil War, and despite presenting an extra large target, he had managed successfully to disperse guerrilla raiders in his district without serious injury to himself. The genteel Southerner won Anna's heart during a shipboard romance while bound for Europe, and their engagement was announced before they docked.

When Queen Victoria got wind of this, she insisted the loving couple be married in London at the Royal Parish of St. Martin-in-the-Fields. This transpired on June 17, 1872. A Canadian pastor, the Reverend Rupert Cochrane, performed the ceremony, and though six foot three inches in height himself, he was dwarfed by the recipients of his blessings. The queen's gifts to the couple included Anna's wedding dress, which incorporated one hundred yards of satin and fifty yards of lace. She also presented the bride with a diamond cluster ring; large gold watches were given to both Anna and Martin. The chain on Anna's watch measured six feet in length. While the couple was in England, many of the country's most eminent physicians examined both of them. Dr. James Simpson of Edinburgh, a famed obstetrician and gynecologist and pioneer in the use of chloroform anaesthesia, declared Anna to be fit, with healthy organs, though proportionately enlarged to her great stature.

The world's largest married couple spent an extended honeymoon visiting the crowned heads of Europe. Their joy was marred by the birth of a stillborn female child in 1872. The infant weighed eighteen pounds at birth, and was reported to measure twenty-seven inches in length. The body was donated to the London Hospital for educational purposes, but apparently it was lost. (My own attempts to track it down by contacting the hospital were fruitless.)

Martin and Anna subsequently settled in the small town of Seville, Ohio, attracted by its lovely rural setting. Their custom-built home had fourteen-foot ceilings, and normal-sized dinner guests had to mount the rungs of the dining-room chairs to obtain a seat. The couple were avid churchgoers. Anna began teaching Sunday school at the First Baptist Church, and a special oversized pew was constructed to accommodate the new parishioners. Amiable and kind, the giants soon became popular and well-liked members of the community, though some altercations did arise from Martin's habit of continuing to wear his Confederate captain's uniform in a northern state, long after the Civil War was over. Children were always welcome in the couple's home, and they especially adored Anna's pet monkey, Buttons. Houseguests included circus friends, among them the Dog Faced Boy, the Skeleton Man and Mrs. Tom Thumb. Perhaps the most unusual of the many visitors was the "Two-Headed Nightingale," actually a pair of Siamese or conjoined twins noted for their beautiful vocal duets, who had also attended the couple's wedding. The cost of the Bates's new home was somewhat more than anticipated and this resulted in another tour, this time with the W.W. Cole Circus, as "The Tallest Couple on the Globe."

On January 19, 1879, tragedy struck once more with the birth of a second child, a twenty-three-pound boy. He lived only eleven hours and is listed in the *Guinness Book of World Records* as the largest baby ever born. *The Medical Record*, a journal of the time, adds that the infant was thirty inches long, had a chest diameter of twenty-four inches and a head circumference of nineteen inches. His feet were five and a half inches long and his breech twenty-seven inches in diameter. Attended initially by Dr. A. P. Beach, Anna had a thirty-six-hour labour with failure to progress. Apparently she passed an estimated six gallons of fluid when her membranes ruptured, a volume attributed by her doctor partly to her large size and partly to generalized "dropsy," or edema. Subsequently the head emerged, but no further progress occurred. This was probably due to shoulder dystocia, when the shoulders become trapped in the birth canal. Dr. Beach attempted to apply forceps, but was unable to find a pair big enough for the infant's head, which lay in a vagina "measuring twelve inches in its posterior aspect and seven to nine inches in its anterior" (or about double the normal dimensions). He summoned Dr. J. D. Robinson from a nearby town to assist, and the two managed to accomplish delivery by using a bandage wrapped around the neck of the baby for traction.

Anna never recovered completely and became quite fatigued in her later years, eventually giving up teaching her beloved Sunday school class. Unfortunately, her medical records have been lost, but it is said that she suffered from "consumption" or tuberculosis, a condition which killed many in her family. The giantess died on August 5, 1888, only a day before her forty-second birthday, apparently peacefully and in her sleep. Her last attending physician, Dr. Beach, listed the cause of death as "heart failure."

Martin had a fifteen-foot memorial erected for Anna in Mound Hill Cemetery, not far from the family homestead. The funeral unfortunately was delayed due to failure to obtain an appropriate sized casket. The undertaker who received the initial order thought someone was a playing a joke on him and sent a standard-sized coffin instead. To avoid a repeat of this incident, Martin ordered his own casket shortly afterwards, apparently not expecting to much outlive his beloved Anna. He survived, however, to the ripe age of seventy-four, and the coffin sat propped against a wall in his barn for many years.

The giant widower did remarry at about the turn of the century, this time to a woman who was just over five feet tall. Anna's great-great-nephew, Dale Swan, told me that the ladies of the church tried to delicately dissuade the prospective bride from the union, because of certain "potential anatomical complications." These did not seem to materialize, or at least if they did it is not recorded, and the couple lived for many years as husband and wife.

Medically, it seems evident that Anna Swan suffered early in life from the effects of excess growth hormone, probably secondary to a pituitary adenoma, a type of brain tumour which affects glandular function. The normal size of her parents and siblings would make a genetic cause for her stature unlikely. The giantess was also well documented to have a goitre, which appears in about one-fourth of such patients. Diabetes, or at least abnormal glucose tolerance is common in this condition and could have contributed to the large size of Anna's babies, as well as to the hydramnios, or large quantity of amniotic fluid found in her pregnancy. This in turn could have been responsible for the failure of her second labour to progress, due to overdistension of the uterine muscles. Growth hormone does cross the placenta and would be the main cause for the huge size of Anna's babies.

High blood pressure is often found with growth hormone excess, and this, combined with diabetes, may have predisposed Anna to pregnancy-induced hypertension, or toxemia. This is often associated with maternal edema (or "dropsy" as described by Dr. Beach); together with the higher infant mortality found with diabetes, it may well have been the reason for Anna's inability to produce healthy infants. Of course, neonatal asphyxia (lack of oxygen) and birth trauma may have played a role in the death of her second offspring, judging from the description of the labour.

Anna's exceptionally difficult labour and the weakness and fatigue she experienced after her second pregnancy lead me to speculate that she may have developed Sheehan's Syndrome, or postpartum necrosis of the pituitary gland. Her abnormal pituitary would have been especially prone to damage from the tumultuous birth. The cause of her death was listed as heart failure, and this is indeed increased in incidence with gigantism. But if Sheehan's Syndrome were present, then the loss of glandular function, especially thyroid and adrenal, would neatly explain Anna's postpartum deterioration and eventual demise. Further light might be shed on her health if records could be found, though that seems unlikely as this late date.

Though it was reported that Anna had tuberculosis, this probably did not cause her death. Dr. Beach would have been very familiar with this condition, which was rampant in the nineteenth century, and would surely have listed it as the cause of death, rather than heart failure. Sheehan's Syndrome, however, would have been difficult to diagnose without modern lab tests which were unavailable at the time.

Anna Swan's medical condition brought her fame and a degree of financial reward, but she must at times have longed to be normal in size. We should remember her, not just for her extraordinary height, but for her dignity and her devotion to her husband and to her community.

George Burden

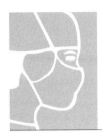

DR. DANIEL HALE WILLIAMS
THE FIRST HEART SURGEON

"Sewed up his heart!" shouted the headline. Readers of a Chicago newspaper gasped at the exciting news, and why not? In 1893, this was a medical miracle made even more newsworthy because it had been performed by one of North America's few black surgeons.

Dr. Daniel Hale Williams was the remarkable surgeon who was clearly committed to defying the status quo of late-nineteenth and early-twentieth-century medicine.

What is significant for Canadians to know is that this man had an ancestral link to the Maritimes. Helen Buckler, in her excellent biography, *Daniel Hale Williams: Negro Surgeon*, traced his heritage, on his mother's side of the family, back to a freed slave who lived in Yarmouth, Nova Scotia, in the late 1700s.

Born in 1856 to Pennsylvania parents of mixed Shawnee Indian, Welsh, Irish, Scottish and African-American blood, Dan was fair-skinned with red hair. Like his parents and grandparents, he took great pride in the knowledge that he could claim African roots. During his lifetime, despite his fair skin, he refused to pass himself off as a white man. This strength of character is not surprising, since, in order to reach his goal of excelling in the medical profession, he was forced to deal with enormous obstacles.

He was only eleven when his father died, and his mother arranged for him to become a shoemaker's apprentice. He hated the tedious work and courageously ran away, making his way back home only to discover that his widowed mother had moved, leaving him to fend for himself.

Dan, however, was not your average youngster. By the age of seventeen, he owned a small barbershop in a town in Wisconsin. Not content with this role, he joined an established business in a nearby community.

Barbering part time, playing the bass fiddle in the evening, Dan was able to earn enough money to pay for private tutoring. After completing high school, he began to read law books, but concluded the legal profession was not for him, especially as he abhorred confrontation.

Several articles in the community's small weekly newspaper caught Dan's attention. They chronicled the interesting adventures of the town's doctor and former mayor, Dr. Henry Palmer. The stories intrigued Dan, and in 1878 he convinced Dr. Palmer to accept him as an apprentice. The next two years proved to be anything but adventurous for the young apprentice. He had to balance mundane duties such as sweeping the doctor's waiting room and cleaning his horse barn with the responsibility of helping to dress wounds, set fractures and test urine samples.

Dan was ecstatic when in 1880 his mentor informed him that he would be prepared to give him the credentials needed for medical school. Elated by this prospect, Dan chose the Chicago Medical College, which was later affiliated with Northwestern University. The young man's first year at medical school proved to be another difficult time in his life. He was barely able to exist on borrowed money, and although he studied constantly, his grades were mediocre. Fortunately, his second year was more rewarding. He found anatomy classes fascinating and was able to visit Mercy Hospital, where he witnessed the impact that Joseph Lister's evolutionary theories on antisepsis were having on surgery.

In March 1883, Daniel Hale Williams was qualified to write MD after his name. Now twenty-seven and equipped with an Illinois medical licence, he opened his office in an area of Chicago that would offer him access to both white and black patients. Dr. Williams soon found himself performing surgery on a regular basis; he was asked to demonstrate his surgical ability to medical students, and his name often appeared in *The Conservator*, a Negro newspaper.

The outstanding surgeon's reputation quickly spread, and he was invited to join the prestigious Hamilton Club, a Republican organization with few black members. He was also appointed to the Illinois State Board of Health, though he was never fully recognized there.

In 1890, a plea for help from a pastor at a local black church served as a cruel reminder of the rampant racism of the day. The Reverend Louis Reynolds was angry that his well-educated sister Emma could not find a

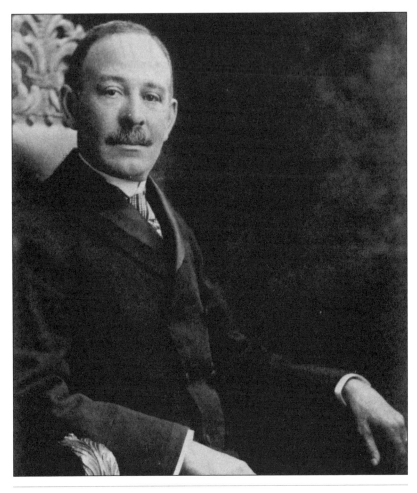

Daniel Hale Williams, chief surgeon at the Freedmen's Hospital, Washington, DC, 1894-1898. *DANIEL HALE WILLIAMS: NEGRO SURGEON*

nursing school that would accept her as a student. Dr. Williams — greatly disturbed by this situation — decided it was time to found a hospital where black doctors could serve as interns and where black women could train as nurses. He insisted on only one thing: it must be an interracial institution that would be open to all, regardless of race, gender or creed. In May

1891, Provident Hospital opened its doors with black and white doctors on staff, and seven young women, including Emma Reynolds, enrolled in the first interracial nursing class in the United States. (A Canadian woman, Jessie Sleet, was a member of that class. She became the first black woman to work as a district nurse for a charitable organization in New York City.)

It was at the new hospital, two years later, that Dr. Williams performed his miraculous surgery. James Cornish was in critical condition when he was rushed to Provident Hospital. He had been stabbed in the chest, was in severe pain and obviously dying. Most colleagues, when faced with such a terrible injury, would not have considered operating. Dr. Williams did not share this kind of reticence. Boldly and skillfully, he repaired the tear in his patient's heart. Today, the significance of this surgery continues to be challenged, but there is little doubt that Dan Williams deserves full credit for performing the first operation of its kind in medical history.

James Cornish made a rapid recovery. The positive outcome encouraged Dr. Williams to perform at least two other successful heart operations. Later, while working at the Freedmen's Hospital in Washington, D.C., he operated on a number of other complex cases. During his time there, fewer than ten postoperative deaths were reported, yet he was never invited to join the District Medical Society, which was a predominantly white professional association. Dr. Williams felt it was imperative that he respond to this racial prejudice. In 1895, with the support of three white and five black physicians, the Medico-Surgical Society of the District of Columbia was formed. The same year, he helped found the National Medical Foundation.

Engrossed in his surgical practice, Williams was shocked to learn that his status at Freedmen's Hospital was being undermined. When the situation became unbearable, he concluded he had no choice but to resign from the hospital and return to his practice in Chicago.

Within months of his return to Chicago, Dr. Williams turned his attention to the South, where he knew the black population desperately needed access to proper medical care. For some time, a medical college in the southern United States had been trying to create an academic environment that would lead to the graduation of a greater number of black doctors. Dr Williams was more than willing to help them achieve this objective. Without remuneration, he began to work and teach at the college. His enormous commitment to improve medical care for blacks living in the American South had a significant payoff: it fostered forty hospitals in twenty different states. Helen Buckler insists that his fervour, his unremitting labour and uncompromising perfectionism truly earned him the right to be known as the "Moses to Negro Medicine."

In 1912, Dr. Williams reluctantly resigned from Provident, the hospital that he had helped found. The man who had replaced him as its medical director had always resented the older physician's high standing in mainstream medicine and had done everything possible to destroy his credibility. However, Dr. Williams' reputation remained unblemished. In 1913, he was the only black man among a hundred surgeons who were formally installed as members of the newly formed American College of Surgeons, and in 1919, black doctors practicing in Missouri presented him with a silver cup to express their appreciation for his work in advancing the medical profession in that state and all of the United States.

On August 4, 1931, Daniel Hale Williams died. In his will, the bulk of his estate was designated for the benefit of his race. The largest bequest, $8,000, went to the National Association for the Advancement of Colored People.

Sadly, the hospital Dr. Williams founded had a troubled existence, even though a new faculty with three hundred beds was opened in 1983. However, this rejuvenation was brief. Five years later, serious financial and management problems resulted in the sudden closure of Provident Hospital. In 1991, the then-derelict facility was purchased by the city, and more than fifty-eight million dollars was spent on renovations. Calls to Provident Hospital in Cook County revealed that there is little evidence at the refurbished facility to mark Dr. Williams's contribution to the original hospital, and there is no official acknowledgment of his remarkable medical career. No play or movie has been made about this extraordinary doctor and surgical pioneer; Helen Buckler's book stands alone.

This raises a question: If Dr. Williams had been white, or if he had chosen to keep his black heritage a secret, would his memory have received the tribute it deserves?

Dorothy Grant

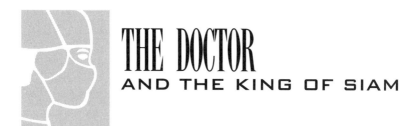

THE DOCTOR
AND THE KING OF SIAM

Most people are familiar with Anna Leonowens, the Victorian-era governess and teacher of the multitudinous offspring of Mongkut, the King of Siam. Anna's book, *The English Governess at the Siamese Court,* created a sensation in the nineteenth century. Her renown was further magnified by Margaret Landon's 1944 biography, *Anna and the King of Siam,* which inspired the subsequent hit musical and Hollywood film, *The King and I.* Few know that after her adventures in Southeast Asia, she moved to Canada, where she spent most of her life. Fewer still realize that beginning with her grandson, James Fyshe, she founded a medical dynasty, all of them McGill graduates with a taste for adventure as strong as her own. (Though Boris Karloff is also a descendant of Anna, we won't include him as he only *played* Dr. Frankenstein's very famous patient.)

Dr. James Fyshe was born in Halifax, Nova Scotia, on March 8, 1879, the first of six siblings. His father, Thomas Fyshe, was an executive with the Bank of Nova Scotia, and he had married Anna's daughter Avis in June of the previous year in New York. James was something of a favourite with his grandmother, who shared their Halifax home. His childhood was dominated by this strong-willed woman who regaled him with stories of her adventures in India, Thailand, Russia and other exotic places. Her tutelage was strict, with little time allowed away from schooling and homework. Despite this, his childhood diary indicates James's lively interest in ponds and trout fishing, proving at least an occasional escape from his grandmother's watchful eye.

In 1888, Anna packed up the entire clan, except the children's poor father, Thomas, for a five-year sojourn in Germany. This was arranged to further her grandchildren's education and to allow her to attend lectures

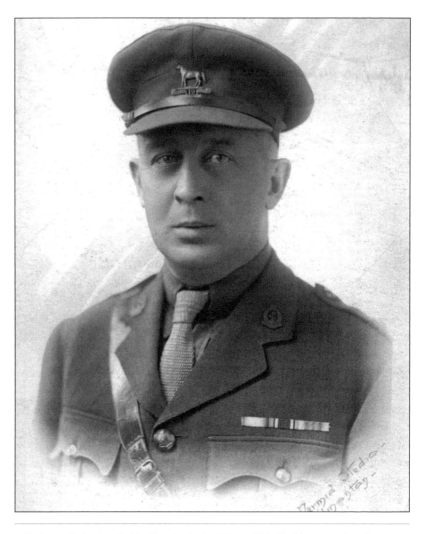

Dr. James Fyshe travelled to Siam in the footsteps of his illustrious grandmother, Anna Leonowens. THE FYSHE FAMILY

on Sanskrit (apparently a waste of time as she turned out to know more Sanskrit than her instructor). While in Europe, she assumed the care of two more grandchildren, offspring of her son Louis, who had become a prosperous businessman in Thailand. Unfortunately, Louis' wife, the daughter of a Thai princess, died in her mid-thirties of kidney disease. So he sent the children off to be raised by their grandmother while he pursued an unconventional lifestyle (at least for a Victorian-era Englishman), which included concubines, a harem and troupes of acrobats, boxers, and dancers.

After the return of his family, now grown in number by two, Thomas, the long-suffering bank executive, was transferred to Montreal. Not long after the family's arrival, Avis died of "acute gastrointestinal catarrh and congestive heart failure," and Anna assumed the duty of raising her eight grandchildren.

James enrolled in Arts at Harvard University, but in 1901 he transferred to McGill, where he earned a BA. By 1904 he decided his future lay in medicine, and he subsequently graduated from McGill Medical School, standing seventh in his class. James did his medical residency at the Montreal General Hospital and afterwards became medical superintendent at the Alexandra Hospital for Contagious Diseases.

He did not remain there long before he decided to follow in his grandmother's footsteps and take up the position of Superintendent of the Government Hospital in Bangkok, as well as the title of Assistant Medical Officer of Health. On his arrival in Bangkok in 1907, after a four-month sea journey, his Uncle Louis greeted Dr. Fyshe with great fanfare. A prim and proper Victorian gentleman, thanks to his grandmother's teachings, James no doubt looked a little askance at his uncle's notorious activities. He was also faced with a formidable task in reforming the Thai health care system and dealing with the myriad diseases endemic in Southeast Asia. Even with King Chulalongkorn as an ally, the bureaucracy of Siam was slow to make changes, which James must have found extremely frustrating. King Chulalongkorn died of kidney disease in 1910 (one wonders if some hereditary form of renal disease, perhaps polycystic kidneys, ran in the royal family). With the loss of his royal patron's support, James realized his task was hopeless. He decided to return to Canada in 1911. However, his stay had not been fruitless. While in Thailand, Dr. Fyshe had gained a young bride, Julia Corisande Mattice, from Montreal, known more commonly by her interesting sobriquet, "Zulu." A son, Thomas, had been born to the couple in 1909, before their departure.

On his return to Montreal, James became superintendent of the Montreal General Hospital. He served as major in World War I and after the war moved to Alberta, where he became administrator of the Royal Alexandra Hospital and helped found the Alberta Hospital Association. James subsequently moved to the small town of Waterhole, near the Peace River. His granddaughter, Dr. Avis Fyshe Boyar, tells me he was the first person to cross the frozen Peace River in a Model T Ford while on a house call. Unfortunately, Dr. James Fyshe died of an apparent heart attack while crossing the street to his clinic in 1921. He was only forty-three.

James's only child, son Thomas, went on to graduate from McGill Medical School in 1936. Dr. Thomas "Tam" Fyshe had worked his way through medical school prospecting in northern Quebec; then — exhibiting the family wanderlust — he went off to Peru to work on top of a mountain as medical officer for a mining company. In order to take his annual leave, Tam Fyshe had to descend 14,000 feet on muleback along the old Inca trail to reach Lima.

He subsequently worked in the Canadian Medical Corps during the Second World War, treating survivors of the Dieppe disaster. Later he served on the front lines in Italy, his arrival only slightly delayed when the troop carrier in which he was travelling was torpedoed and sank.

At the termination of the war, while shipping back to Canada, Tam Fyshe met George Gilmour, the Chancellor of McMaster University, who convinced him to go to work in Hamilton. He agreed and took a position as a general surgeon at the prestigious McGregor Clinic.

During his career, Tam Fyshe worked on an early prototype of the artificial knee and also performed the first open-heart surgery in Hamilton. His daughter, Dr. Avis Fyshe Boyar, describes him as being a very modest man who never considered his first "valve job" as anything especially extraordinary. He passed away, in 1998, at the age of eighty-nine.

Avis is also a McGill graduate, a family physician with a special interest in palliative care. Another victim of the family adventure bug, she served a stint in China, then set up the first palliative care unit of its kind at the King's Hospital in Saudi Arabia, and finally returned to western Canada.

George Burden

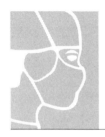

ALEXANDER GRAHAM BELL
MEDICAL INVENTOR

If you asked Alexander Graham Bell his profession, his reply until the day he died would have been, "teacher of the deaf." All of his life he was destined to share an intimate connection with the hearing impaired; his mother became profoundly deaf later in life, and his beloved wife, Mabel, was totally deaf from the age of five, after a bout of scarlet fever. Bell's grandfather was a pioneer of speech therapy, and his father, Alexander Melville Bell, was the inventor of a system called Visible Speech. Visible Speech used a system of symbols to represent the positioning of the palate, mouth and tongue. Even the profoundly deaf could learn to speak by using these symbols. Young Aleck showed early promise in the field of speech therapy; as a child he taught his dog to say a few rudimentary phrases by manipulating the animal's glottis. Later, while living in Brantford, Ontario, he learned to speak fluently with the neighbouring Mohawk Indians using the Visible Speech system of his father. As a result, they initiated him into the tribe with full ceremonies.

Aleck Bell was born in Edinburgh, Scotland, on March 3, 1847. Later his family lived in London, but after his two brothers contracted tuberculosis and died, young Aleck began to ail, and his father decided to flee the London smog for the fresh air of Upper Canada, where Aleck thrived. Later he moved to Boston to teach the hearing impaired. There he fell in love with and married one of his students, Mabel Hubbard, who encouraged her husband in all of his endeavours.

At the age of twenty-nine, he invented and patented the telephone. This marked not the culmination but rather the beginning of his long and diverse career as an inventor. While his permanent home became Washington, D.C., Bell loathed the hot, humid summers and subsequently

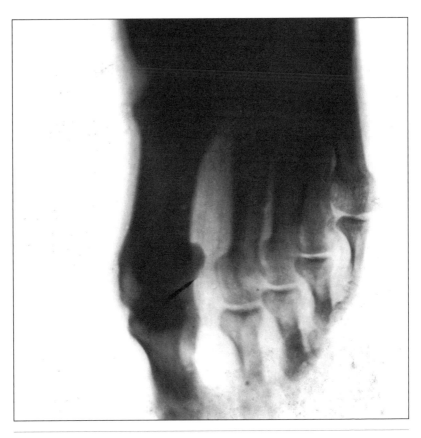

The first medical X-ray in Canada. Taken by Dr. Alexander Graham Bell, this film allowed doctors to find and remove a needle from the long-suffering patient's foot. PARKS CANADA / ALEXANDER GRAHAM BELL NATIONAL HISTORIC SITE

built a large house on his estate on Bras d'Or Lake in Cape Breton. Beinn Bhreagh, meaning "beautiful mountain" in Gaelic, remains a home of Bell's descendants to this day. It witnessed the fruition of some of Alexander Bell's most innovative ideas. These included many medical devices, the first powered flight in the British Empire and pioneering work in hydroplane technology, which was to set world records for speed in water craft.

When American President James Garfield was shot in 1881, his physicians asked Bell to locate the bullet. Bell hoped to use a metal detector, which he had developed, to carry out this task. Though previously successful, the device malfunctioned due to the failure to remove all metal from the hospital room as Bell had requested. The mattress on which the President rested contained metal coils, so new an innovation at the time that few had heard of it. Bell rushed back to his lab and developed a "bullet probe" or "telephonic needle probe" which could be inserted into the entry wound. This invention was used very effectively in the Boer War and in World War I, but it was unfortunately too late to aid President Garfield. Ironically, the bullet was found in a fairly innocuous location at the autopsy, and it is thought that death probably resulted from infection due to repeated manual probing by the President's doctors. Bell was later awarded an Honorary Doctorate of Medicine at Heidelberg University for his bullet probe.

Another medical device invented by Bell was the audiometer. Developed in 1879, it is similar to the ones we use today to assess hearing loss. In honour of his work in this field, the unit by which we measure sound, the decibel, was named for the inventor. Genetics was another area Bell explored, and he studied in depth the patterns of deafness and longevity in humans.

Bell became fascinated by Wilhelm Conrad Roentgen's invention of the X-ray in 1895 and began working on his own device, taking the first medical X-ray in Canada at his home in Baddeck, in October 1897. True to the inventor's practical nature, the subject was not merely a healthy volunteer but a man with persistent foot and leg pain. Two local physicians, Dr. MacDonald and Dr. McKeen, asked Bell's help in locating a broken needle fragment in this patient's foot. The X-ray showed the needle clearly, and the doctors removed it, completely relieving the man's suffering. Bell also was the first person in North America to advocate treatment of deep-seated cancers using radium encased in glass tubes, thus becoming our first radiation oncologist.

Bell became interested in respiratory disease after it claimed the life of one of his sons. He invented an artificial lung, the "vacuum jacket," remarkably like the iron lung used fifty years later to save polio victims. He hoped also to use this to resuscitate victims of drowning and successfully employed it to revive a sheep which had drowned. One of Bell's

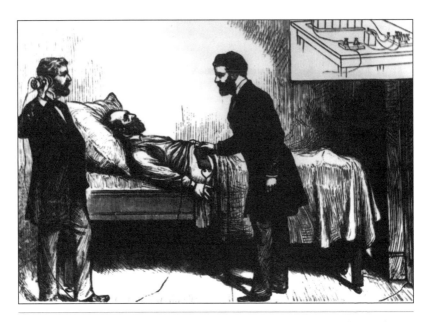

Dr. Alexander Graham Bell searching with his metal detector for the bullet which felled American President James Garfield. PARKS CANADA / ALEXANDER GRAHAM BELL NATIONAL HISTORIC SITE

employees witnessed this and, convinced it was the work of the devil, quit his job and even refused to accept a final paycheque.

Though his amiable nature made him well loved in the community, Bell had developed a bit of a reputation as an eccentric among some of the people in Baddeck. His early aviation experiments with huge kites did nothing to dispel this reputation, nor did his tendency to run around outside in his bathing suit during storms or float on Bras d'Or Lake on an inner tube smoking cigars for hours on end. Even after dark, his granddaughter reminisced, she'd often spot the glowing tip of his cigar in the gloom of the inlet.

Shortly after the Wright brothers' first flight, Bell formed the Aerial Experimentation Association. Under his auspices, John McCurdy designed and piloted the first heavier-than-air aircraft in the British Empire. The Silver Dart lifted off from the ice in Baddeck on January 9, 1909, flying nearly a mile at an altitude of thirty feet. This technology was subsequently adapted to build high-speed hydrofoils (or hydrodromes, as Bell called them). It was hoped these vessels could be used to hunt down German U-Boats that were causing such devastation to shipping in World War I. In 1919, together with Casey Baldwin, Bell set the world water-speed record of 70.86 miles per hour in the HD 4. This record was not broken for ten years. With the end of the war, the government lost interest in the hydrodrome project. The work of Bell and Baldwin was revived in the 1970s when Canada built a hydrofoil submarine chaser, appropriately named the *Bras d'Or*.

The HD 4 rotted on the shore for years until salvaged and incorporated into the displays of the Alexander Graham Bell Museum in Baddeck. This national historic site retains many of Bell's original inventions, which were donated by the family, as well as a full-scale replica of the HD 4. Here also can be seen Bell's artificial lung and his early X-ray equipment. There is even a telephone which used sunlight to transmit sound, impractical at the time, but anticipating fibre-optic and laser communication by a hundred years.

Aleck Bell loved to invent, and he loved people. One of his employees had eight children and did not own a house. The man was astounded when Bell handed him an envelope containing the deed to a home as a Christmas present. Perhaps most of all, the inventor adored children. Bell met Helen Keller when she was only six years old, and, recognizing the child's potential, he directed her to the Perkins Institute, where she came under the tutelage of Annie Sullivan. Later in life, Keller dedicated her autobiography to Bell to thank him for the help he had given her.

Bell was financially impractical, but his wife and friends ensured that he had the means to continue to invent and to indulge his generous dedication to science and humanity. However, he never allowed any of his medical devices to be patented as he felt it immoral to benefit financially from the misfortune of others. The inventor died at Beinn Breagh in 1922, and his wife followed five months later. Here they lie buried, their graves overlooking the misty inlets of Cape Breton which they loved so much.

George Burden

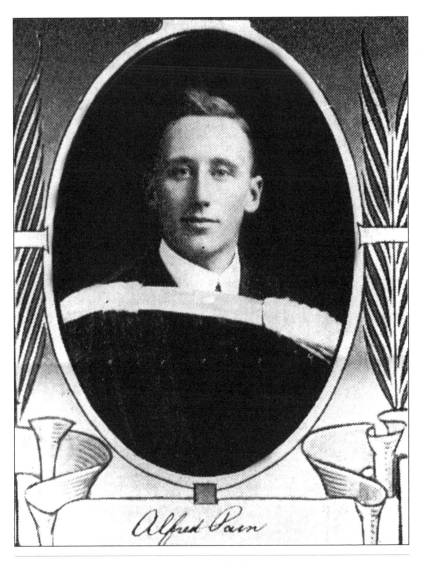

Dr. Alfred Pain, a second-class passenger on the *Titanic*. COURTESY OF ALAN HUSTAK COLLECTION

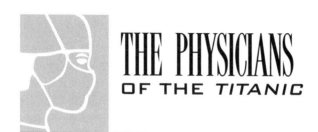

THE PHYSICIANS
OF THE *TITANIC*

Millions of words have been written about the sinking of the *Titanic* on April 15, 1912. Despite the monumental effort to try to make some sense of this horrendous tragedy, countless mysteries and thousands of untold stories of those who survived and those who did not continue to interest researchers.

For me, the nine doctors, eight men and one woman, now known to have been on that ill-fated ship represent a most fascinating conundrum. Although several of these physicians have received some attention, others remain notable only because they had the bad luck of being on the *Titanic* when it met its infamous demise.

Dr. William O'Loughlin was the White Star Line's chief surgeon. Born in Ireland, he was an orphan who was raised and educated by an uncle. He proved to be a distinguished student and in 1869 should have received a medical degree. But this didn't happen. Unfortunately for him, the Catholic university he had attended did not have a royal charter that would enable it to grant this kind of academic recognition. O'Loughlin, a devout Catholic, had refused to attend Trinity College, a Protestant university. This dogmatic stance cost him the chance to earn a medical degree. Instead, he received only a license to practise medicine, although subsequently he did become a licentiate of the King's and Queen's College of Physicians in Ireland.

Dr. O'Loughlin, who never married, had a passion for the sea. Ironically, he once declared that when he died he wanted his body thrown into the sea, which for him must have represented the "mistress" he loved very much.

Dr. O'Loughlin's first responsibility, prior to the *Titanic*'s sailing, was to examine the crew and steerage passengers. His assistant, Dr. J. Edward Simpson, joined him in this important task. Heads were scrutinized for lice, and the doctors were also on the lookout for infectious diseases such as tuberculosis and trachoma, a highly infectious and potentially blinding disease of the eye. Any passenger with trachoma was unceremoniously ordered off the ship, since American immigration laws did not permit them to enter the country.

Dr. J. Edward Simpson, the assistant surgeon, was also Irish. Born in Belfast, he was the son of a doctor. He studied at the Royal University of Ireland, and unlike O'Loughlin, he did earn a medical degree from Queen's University in Belfast. He was a member of the British Medical Association. Only thirty-seven at the time of the disaster, he was a married man and the father of a young son. Apparently, it was his poor health that had influenced him to pursue a "healthy" career at sea, and this decision led to his serving as a medical officer on several steamships.

The *Titanic*'s reign at sea lasted only a few days, and during this brief period of glory, its passengers experienced few noteworthy medical problems. One lady, who was a first class passenger, fell down a flight of stairs, breaking a small bone in her arm. One account reports that her arm was placed in a plaster cast by Dr. Simpson. Another states that she was treated by Dr. Henry Frauenthal, a distinguished orthopedic surgeon who was also a passenger on the ship.

Dr. Frauenthal was the founder of the New York Hospital for Joint Diseases. Born in Pennsylvania, he had a background in analytical chemistry, and he studied medicine at Bellevue Hospital Medical Clinic. Early in his medical career he became convinced that a hospital devoted entirely to chronic joint diseases was desperately needed. In 1904, he opened a small clinic. On the first day only eight patients were treated, but by the end of that year it had provided almost ten thousand treatments. Dr. Frauenthal quickly earned a reputation as an outstanding specialist, and during the same time he acquired a sizeable fortune. He, along with his new bride and his brother, were first-class passengers on the *Titanic*.

Dr. Alfred Pain was also a passenger on the ship. The young University of Toronto Medical School graduate was travelling in second-class accommodations. Born in Hamilton, Ontario, he had been an excellent student and a fine athlete. After spending a short time as a house doctor at the Hamilton City Hospital, he had gone to England to further his studies. Originally, he hoped to finance his journey home by finding a position as a ship's doctor. When this couldn't be arranged, he booked passage on the doomed *Titanic*.

Dr. William Minahan, a graduate of Rush Medical College, Chicago, was the third member of his family to enter the medical profession. In 1899, he established a practice in Fond du Lac, Wisconsin, where he became a highly respected physician, well known not only for his surgical skills but also for the large amount of charity work he did. A first-class passenger, forty-four-year old Dr. Minahan was travelling with his wife, Lillian, and his sister.

Dr. Ernest Moraweck, an internationally known eye specialist, was a resident of Frankfort, Kentucky. A widower, he was returning home from medical business in Europe. He assisted a fellow passenger by removing a foreign body from her eye.

Dr. Alice Leader, a fifty-five-year-old physician, practised medicine in New York with her husband, John. A first-class passenger, she shared a cabin with another woman.

Dr. Washington Dodge, also a first-class passenger, graduated from the University of California medical school sometime in the mid-1880s. In 1896, he left the medical profession and entered politics. Apparently he did extremely well in his new role and had become a very popular and affluent member of the political community in San Francisco. He and his second wife and their five-year-old son, Washington Dodge, Jr., were on their way home from a visit to Paris. They had been in Europe primarily for him to consider a prestigious position with an international banking firm. The doctor's health seems to have been failing, and during his time in Paris he had consulted a specialist.

Almost nothing is known about Dr. Arthur Brewe, a physician from Philadelphia.

On April 14, 1912, all of the physicians on the *Titanic* must have spent the early evening hours feeling entirely safe aboard the majestic ocean liner. Early in the day, Dr. O'Loughlin had lunched with Tommy Andrews, the proud builder of the ship. That evening, his dinner companion was Bruce Ismay, the Managing Director of the White Star Line, the company that had audaciously built what it contended was a "practically unsinkable" ship. The fanciful deception was about to be shattered.

"Iceberg, right ahead!" cried the lookout high up in the *Titanic*'s crow's-nest. It was approximately eleven-forty p.m. on Sunday, April 14, 1912. For many of the ship's crew and its passengers, these words would soon translate into a death knell.

At the time of the collision, Dr. William O'Loughlin was probably asleep in what stewardess Violet Jessop described in her memoirs as his "magnificently appointed cabin." He must have recognized very quickly that the ship was in real danger. Mary Sloan, another stewardess, encountered him soon after the collision. She asked if he knew what was happening. His words were far from reassuring: "Child, things are very bad."

It seems that he was on his way to see a passenger, Mrs. Henry Harper, on D deck, who had requested that he visit her cabin because she wanted him to convince her ill husband that he was too sick to get out of bed. Looking sombre, the physician passed on the bad news to the couple. "They tell me that trunks are floating around in the hold; you may as well go on deck." His next movements are hard to trace, but a number of people remembered seeing him in the company of several crew members as well as with Dr. Simpson.

Around two a.m., shortly before the *Titanic*'s fate was sealed forever, one of the ship's bakers discovered Dr. O'Loughlin rummaging through a pantry on B deck, the deck directly above the ship's hospital. Apparently, not long after the last lifeboat had left the sinking ship, the physician had declared that he would meet his end indoors. He said he refused to die in freezing water surrounded by others enduring the same terrible fate. Instead, he had gone to the pantry looking for whiskey to dull his senses. He knew that when the ship reached a certain depth, his lungs would implode. "Not necessarily painless, but it has the advantage of being quick."

Dr. O'Loughlin was eulogized as a true hero and a physician to whom "it made no difference whether the call came from a poor immigrant in steerage or a millionaire in the Royal Suite." A memorial fund in his memory was established at Saint Vincent's Hospital in New York, an institution he had generously supported. He also received, posthumously, the American Medicine Gold Medal Award.

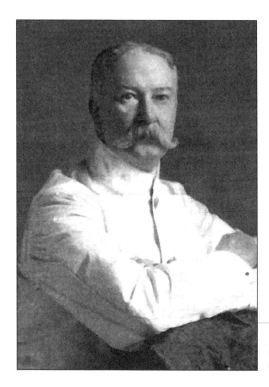

Dr. William O'Loughlin, senior surgeon on the *Titanic*.
ENCYCLOPEDIA TITANICA

Dr. Simpson also lost his life in the sinking, and he, too, has gone down in the disaster's history as a hero. Not only is he remembered as a very brave man but also as an Irishman who met death true to his heritage. Mary Sloan and another stewardess met him during the confusion that followed the collision with the iceberg. They both liked him because he had a marvellous sense of humour. This time there was nothing amusing about the situation, but Dr. Simpson, realizing the women were very frightened, led them to a nearby dispensary, where he poured each of them a glass of whiskey. When Mary asked him if he thought she would need the alcoholic beverage, he replied, "You might need it later on." Hearing these words, the other stewardess began to weep. Mary, however, insisted that she was not afraid. Simpson's response was to raise his glass and exclaim, "Spoken like a true Ulster woman!" His body, if it was recovered, was never identified, although one writer claims that Simpson's medical bag was salvaged from the wreck.

Charles H. Lightoller, the Second Officer on the *Titanic*, miraculously survived the sinking. During his appearance at a board of inquiry, he vividly recalled a brief encounter he had had with doctors O'Loughlin and Simpson. He reported that they obviously knew the score and were "still assisting by showing a calm and cool exterior to the passengers." Each of them had come up to him to shake his hand and say goodbye.

Survivors later reported that the conduct of the physicians on board had been exemplary, that they actively assisted passengers and had refused seats in the lifeboats. Only one of them will forever have shame associated with his name. He was Dr. Frauenthal, the noted orthopedic surgeon from New York. In a dramatic declaration of love for his wife, who had found a place in a lifeboat, he had screamed, "I cannot leave you." Then, to the utter disgust of one of the crew members, he and his brother suddenly jumped into the vessel. Some say that Dr. Frauenthal was the bulky man who landed on a lady passenger, breaking two of her ribs. Ironically, fifteen years later, in 1927, Dr. Frauenthal committed suicide by jumping out of the seventh floor of his apartment building in New York. The medical examiner assigned to the case attributed his death to "a fall from a window due to mental derangement."

Even more bizarre were the terms of Frauenthal's will. He ordered that he be cremated and his ashes stored in the Hospital for Joint Diseases that he had founded until the fiftieth anniversary of the hospital's incorporation. On that day, he requested his ashes be scattered from the roof "to the four winds." This was done on October 5, 1955.

Dr. Alfred Pain, the youthful physician born in Hamilton, Ontario, had befriended a young Canadian woman he had met during the cruise. He made a point of finding her and encouraged her to hurry to find a place in a lifeboat. Later, learning of his death, she was heartbroken that she hadn't taken the time to say goodbye. Tearfully, she explained that she had failed to do this because she believed the *Titanic* was "unsinkable" and that she would soon see him again.

"Be brave. No matter what happens, be brave!" were Dr. William Minahan's last words to his wife as he helped her into lifeboat number four. The Wisconsin doctor's body was identified by his personal effects, including a clinical thermometer. When news of his death reached his colleagues, they had only positive things to say about him. "Dr. Minahan was an untiring student, a clever diagnostician, a kind physician and a wonderfully pleasing man socially."

Dr. Ernest Moraweck from Kentucky also perished. The young lady who had dined with him the evening before the sinking had passed him on her way to the lifeboats. Dr. Moraweck told her he was trying to find out what was happening. He was never seen again.

Dr. Alice Leader from New York City was among the twenty-eight people who found safety in lifeboat number eight. Three crewmen had managed to join the twenty-five women on the boat, allegedly to serve as oarsmen. To Dr. Leader's great concern, it was quickly discovered that "none of the seamen knew their place." In fact, one of the women had to tell a steward to put an oar in the oarlock. "Do you put it in that hole?" he asked. "Certainly," she replied. Dr. Leader practised medicine in New York for another twenty years. She died in Florida on April 27, 1944.

Dr. Washington Dodge also survived, and on April 19, while still in New York, he published the following message in the *San Francisco Bulletin*: "Please extend through the columns of today's *Bulletin* to all inquiring friends, whose telegrams were handed me aboard the rescuing steamer *Carpathia*, my affectionate greetings and my undying gratitude for their loving messages. My family, thank God, were all saved, being one of the very few where this was the case. As soon as able to resume our Journey, which I trust will be in a few days, I shall start for my beloved city. Sincerely yours, Washington Dodge."

Arthur Brewe, the doctor from Philadelphia, was among the six physicians who lost their lives when the *Titanic* went down.

Not enough is known about most of the physicians who experienced the *Titanic* catastrophe, but we do know the doctors who died in the sinking went to their deaths with dignity and with the clear understanding that they were sacrificing their lives to save others.

Dorothy Grant

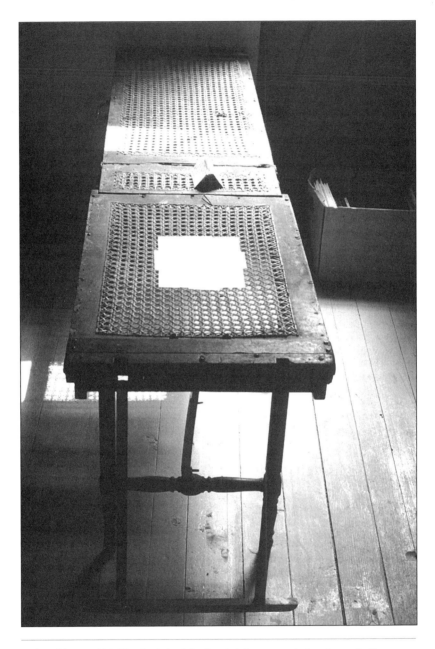

The table on which *Titanic* victim John Jacob Astor was embalmed, now in the collection of the East Hants Historical Museum in Selma, Nova Scotia. GEORGE BURDEN

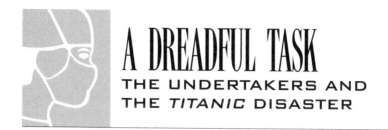

A DREADFUL TASK

THE UNDERTAKERS AND
THE *TITANIC* DISASTER

A chilling announcement appeared in *The Acadian Recorder,* a Halifax newspaper, on April 27, 1912. It stated: "John Snow & Sons have made arrangements whereby all the bodies arriving on Monday aboard the *MacKay-Bennett* will be embalmed by them and their staff, assisted by nearly every embalmer in Nova Scotia, New Brunswick, and Prince Edward Island. The Funeral Directors Association of the Maritime Provinces allow only experienced men and embalmers to become members, and about forty of these members are either in Halifax or on their way there."

In fact, about forty-three undertakers answered the call, and only when they arrived in Halifax would they have begun to comprehend the horrendous task they faced. Even for the most experienced, it must have been heartbreaking to face the devastating task of embalming the many victims of the *Titanic* catastrophe.

In keeping with the male-dominated business world of the time, only two women were included in the group. They were Mrs. Elizabeth Walsh and her sister, Annie O'Neil, from Saint John, New Brunswick, who were considered to be the most appropriate individuals to assume the sensitive responsibility of embalming women's bodies. Mrs. Walsh apparently also embalmed the body of a baby that was among the first to be taken from the sea and the only child that remained unclaimed.

The White Star Line that owned the *Titanic* had arranged to obtain hundreds of caskets from manufacturers all over the Eastern provinces, and Snow & Sons had contacted a coffin company requesting that its staff work night and day to supply a large number of its product. As the coffins arrived in the city, many were taken to the wharves that have nuzzled the edges of Halifax's magnificent harbour for hundreds of years. It was not the first time such grim reminders of death rested on the docks, but never had there been so many destined to become final shelters for bodies recovered from the frigid waters of the Atlantic.

The White Star Line had chartered several vessels to search for victims of the disaster. One of them, the cable ship *MacKay-Bennett*, recovered many bodies found floating in an area that extended over several kilometres surrounding the location where the majestic ship had gone down. In a strange twist of fate, the crew encountered bodies floating together in large numbers. They described the scene as being strangely reminiscent "of witnessing a flock of seagulls in the fog." But unlike seagulls whose liberating wings enable the birds to free themselves from the grasp of a greedy ocean, these were the ship's dead, whose life jackets had kept their doomed bodies rising and falling for several days at the mercy of the waves.

Accompanying the crew on their disheartening recovery mission was "a leading local undertaker, John Snow of Snow & Co." With stoic pragmatism, he had made sure the indispensable accoutrements of his trade had come with him. These items included more than one hundred coffins and huge quantities of embalming fluid. Anticipating that many burials would take place at sea, he had added scrap iron and rolls of canvas to the gloomy inventory. Snow had also insisted that the ship carry more than eighteen thousand kilograms of ice to reduce the chance of further deterioration of those bodies that could not immediately be embalmed.

Some of the bodies recovered were said to be badly disfigured, and it was rumoured that some passengers had sustained terrible injuries as the invading sea viciously assaulted the sinking ship. There has always been considerable debate about the allegations of massive injuries. Yet those who shared personal accounts of seeing many of the bodies generally insisted that most "looked as calm as if they were asleep," and the formal inquiries that followed the tragedy confirmed that most victims had died of exposure.

During its thirteen days at sea, the *MacKay-Bennett* found three hundred and six bodies. One hundred and sixteen of them were buried at sea; this number has been controversial, as it has never been adequately explained how the victims were selected for an ocean burial. One theory is that all of the bodies first retrieved from the Atlantic were handled this way, but this was halted when White Star Line objected to this seemingly callous treatment. Captain Fred Lardner, the master of the vessel, did state that many of these bodies could not be identified, and some of the identified, he claimed, were badly damaged or already in a state of advanced decomposition. Later, when cornered by reporters who demanded better explanations of why the bodies of many crew members and steerage passengers had not been brought back to Halifax, Lardner insisted that his decision had nothing to do with class consciousness. He declared that it had happened because "it was more than his embalmer could handle." The *MacKay-Bennett* did, in fact, run out of embalming fluid and had to obtain an additional supply from another vessel, the *Minia*. However, the captain admitted that "no prominent man was committed to the deep." His reason was that "it seemed wise to embalm the bodies of those identified victims who might have possessed large estates."

The return to Halifax on April 30 was a bittersweet occasion for the *MacKay-Bennett's* crew, who must have been anxious to escape from its cargo of death. Newspapers painted a stark picture of the returning vessel containing many bodies covered by tarpaulins. In one of the ship's holds, they were said to be literally piled "one on top of another." On the Coaling Number 4 dock at HMCS Dockyard, undertakers' carriages were lined up to remove coffins and bodies from the ship. Also waiting at dockside were numerous officials and those identified as next-of-kin or their designated representatives, who had arrived in closed carriages, automobiles and taxicabs.

A reporter for *The Halifax Evening Mail* provided his readers with a scenario of death in its most brutal manifestations. "The first bodies taken ashore were those of the crew. Their bodies had not been embalmed or even sewn up in canvas and presented such a gruesome sight that it would be impossible to picture. The bodies were carried on stretchers by members of the *MacKay-Bennett* crew, and at times as many as thirty or forty bodies were in a heap on deck where they had been taken from the ice-filled hold. The second-class passengers and steerage were sewn up in canvas bags, and they were brought ashore later. They were embalmed and had all been identified. On the wharf, Messrs. Snow & Sons had fully thirty teams, and the bodies were taken away as fast as they could be brought ashore. At 10 a.m., the various hearses began to remove the bodies from the yard." It was a lengthy ordeal to remove and transport all of the bodies from the *MacKay-Bennett*. More than three hours had passed before the macabre job ended with the unloading of the bodies of the first-class passengers, which had all been partially embalmed and placed in coffins.

Because of its location, cold interior and glassed-in areas, the Mayflower Curling Club was chosen to become the crucial facility in the melancholy task of dealing with the recovered bodies. Then located on Agricola Street between McCully and May streets, the club had been subjected to a dramatic transformation. In preparation for the complexities of dealing with the dead, a section of the building was partitioned off to accommodate thirty-four benches, on which the embalmers could perform their sombre ritual of preparing the bodies for burial. Draped in black, the main part of the rink now held close to seventy square frames, two feet high, each large enough to house three coffins. The surrealistic setting was captured graphically in an article that appeared in the Montreal newspaper, *The Gazette*. The account must have horrified readers:

HALIFAX, APRIL 30. Strangely solemn and profoundly impressive is the interior of the Mayflower curling rink, which became a morgue today. This structure, which has on more than one occasion been the scene of all that represents life and gaiety, has been transformed for the silent sleepers gathered from the deep. Never before in the history of Halifax has such a spectacle been witnessed. All this afternoon and tonight more than a score of embalmers with a large number of assistants, were engaged in embalming the bodies at the Mayflower morgue brought in from the scene of the *Titanic* disaster. Orders were given by the White Star Line that all bodies should be embalmed and properly clothed and prepared for burial. The bodies so far examined present no mark of mutilation. Most others are frozen and many slightly decomposed. As a result of the frost, the work of the undertakers has been of necessity retarded.

The embalmers working at the rink focused their attention on identified bodies, while the unidentified were shunted to a temporary holding area. There have been rumours that attempts were made to bribe some undertakers to give priority to certain bodies, but if this did happen, it is believed that the White Star Line summarily put an end to such unethical tactics.

Most of the bodies arrived at the rink with their clothing intact. All garments were removed and catalogued. Forensic science was more primitive then, and it was important to describe every possible clue to someone's identity. Such information came from the undertakers, whose duties involved the intimate aspects of embalming a body. They provided for each victim facts about gender, estimated age and weight, as well as hair colour, scars, birth marks, tattoos, etc. This information became part of a portfolio that included other data, such as the number used on a coffin. In cases where a body would be buried in Halifax, information about its final burial site was noted. Photographs were also taken "where features are at all distinguishable."

The poignant task of addressing many of the logistics associated with dealing with such a large number of dead was said to have taken place in a "very much businesslike" setting. Still, it must have been an incredibly shocking experience for the people who were recruited to make lists of the material goods found on the bodies. It also must have been paradoxical to find oneself handling items that in some cases represented great wealth, and in others the pitiful belongings of passengers and crew members who might possess little more than the clothes on their backs.

Lists of the effects found on the *Titanic's* victims are now an invaluable historical resource housed among the Nova Scotia Public Archives' records in Halifax.

BODY 124. Colonel John Jacob Astor IV, 1st class Passenger. Multi-millionaire, age 47. Light hair and moustache. Blue serge suit; blue handkerchief with 'A.V.'; belt with gold buckle; brown boots with red rubber soles; brown flannel shirt, 'J.J.A.' on back of collar. Gold watch; cuff links, gold with diamonds; diamond ring with three stones; £225 in English notes, $2440 in notes; £5 in gold; 7 shilling in silver; 5 ten franc pieces; gold pencil; pocketbook.

BODY 223, Unidentified Male, probably a steward, age about 20. Height 5 ft. 5 in.; weight 145 lbs. Brown hair. Eye teeth extra long. Wore steward's uniform. No aids to identification.

To help ensure that the families would have the best opportunity to officially identify their deceased loved ones, one end of the Mayflower building, which had previously been used to observe curlers in action, was chosen as a viewing area. There people waited in bewildered anticipation until, following completion of the embalming procedure, the name of a deceased individual was called out. Those recognizing the name would then come forward to be exposed to a painful close view of a body that had just left an embalmer's care. It is impossible to imagine the atmosphere in the rink, as the family members of a deceased person or their official representatives, left their seats and tentatively approached a body. The building must have echoed with their cries as the mourners viewed the corpse of a parent, sibling, close friend or colleague.

Frank Newell, an undertaker from Yarmouth, probably never dreamed that he would also be personally affected by the *Titanic*'s demise. This bizarre event occurred when, during his hard work, he suddenly encountered the body of a relative, A.W. Newell, who had been a first-class passenger on the ship. Apparently overwhelmed by this discovery, the poor fellow collapsed on the floor beside the body. Some say it was his uncle, but this has never been established as fact.

When it became apparent that Halifax would become the centre for dealing with the legal ramifications associated with the *Titanic*'s loss, the provincial government implemented a number of appropriate strategies. In particular, steps were taken to eliminate a bureaucratic nightmare, and two men assumed key roles. They were John Henry Barnstead, who was Halifax's deputy registrar of deaths, and Dr. W.D. Finn, the coroner and medical examiner. Along with their staffs, they established an office above the rink, and this arrangement made it possible for death certificates to be issued with little delay. It also made it easier for those claiming bodies to arrange the transport of caskets to destinations that were often thousands of kilometres away. One of the puzzling mysteries associated with the *Titanic* disaster is the fact that all of the death certificates issued in Halifax during the spring of 1912 have now gone missing.

Of the three hundred and twenty-eight bodies recovered by Canadian vessels, one hundred and sixteen were buried at sea and two hundred and nine were brought back to Halifax. Fifty-nine of those recovered were claimed by relatives and shipped to their home communities. The remaining one hundred and fifty victims are buried in three cemeteries: Fairview Lawn, Mount Olivet and Baron de Hirsch, all in Halifax. This final disposition of the bodies occurred from May 3 to June 12, 1912. Nineteen of the deceased were interred in the Mount Olivet Catholic Cemetery, ten in the Baron de Hirsch Jewish Cemetery, and one hundred and twenty-one in the Fairview Lawn Cemetery. Of these, forty-three remain unidentified (a baby has now been identified).

Many researchers and experts who investigate unnatural deaths today are fascinated by the unsophisticated techniques that were used to identify the bodies recovered from the *Titanic* disaster. For example, they are intrigued that Rabbi M. Walter was given the responsibility of identifying the bodies of those believed to be Jewish. (It has now been discovered that this man was a rabbinical student, not a rabbi.) Apparently, Walter made his determinations primarily on the basis of "a name or a man's appearance." If this was indeed the case, it proved to be an unsatisfactory form of identification, and a number of people identified by him as Jewish proved to be Catholics, including an Irish fellow from Galway. A number of Italian victims, who most probably were of the Catholic faith, now occupy gravesites in Fairview Lawn Cemetery, primarily a cemetery for Protestants. And for unexplained reasons, some pertinent clues, such as initials found on the clothing of several victims, were overlooked or ignored. But ninety years after the terrible ocean tragedy took place, it is unfair surely to criticize or try to second guess the excruciating identification process that occurred in Halifax during the spring of 1912.

Though the world has had a long-standing and intense fascination with the fate of the *Titanic*, the ship has been a more immediate and formidable presence for Atlantic Canadians. As I walked through the ice and snow in the Fairview Lawn Cemetery near a busy intersection in Halifax's north end, I shuddered, not so much from the cold as from the thought of that terrible day in May, 1912, when thirty-six numbered coffins holding the bodies of *Titanic* victims were laid side-by-side in a common grave in this cemetery. It is not humanly possible to attempt to recapture the sombre, surrealistic setting that must have enveloped the eight hundred or more people who witnessed the mass burial.

I stop to reflect on the inscriptions carved on many of the headstones. Some families of the *Titanic* victims have replaced original grave markers with more elaborate monuments, but class distinction matters little to the dead. Perhaps most pathetic are the simple little monuments that bear only numbers, no names. Other gravesites have headstones that identify someone lost on the *Titanic* and also proclaim extraordinary bravery. On one such monument is carved: "Sacred to the memory of Everett Edward Elliott of the heroic crew S.S. *Titanic*, died on duty April 15, 1912 aged 24 years — Each man stood at his post while all the weaker ones went by and showed once more to all the world how Englishmen should die." Another stone nearby simply reads, "Nearer my God to Thee."

In the spring of 1912, Clarence MacKinnon, the principal of the Presbyterian College at Pine Hill, Halifax, made a prediction that has come true. Thinking of the dead, he said, "They shall rest quietly in our midst under the murmuring pines and hemlocks, but their story shall be told to our children and to our children's children."

The gravestones that mark the burial sites of those who lost their lives as a result of the *Titanic's* sinking will forever serve not only as a cruel reminder of human mortality but also of a spiteful ocean that is capable of destroying even the most unsinkable ships and those who so foolishly put their trust in them.

Dorothy Grant

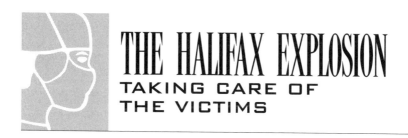

THE HALIFAX EXPLOSION
TAKING CARE OF
THE VICTIMS

It claimed almost three times as many victims as the Great Chicago Fire and the San Francisco earthquake of 1906 combined. Until the advent of the atomic bomb, the Halifax Explosion of December 6, 1917, was the largest man-made detonation ever recorded, and it resulted from the collision of two vessels in Halifax Harbour. It was the height of the First World War, and Halifax was a beehive of activity, shipping munitions, goods and soldiers to England and beleaguered European nations. The Belgian relief ship *Imo* was exiting the Bedford Basin early that cool, clear December morning when — through a series of piloting errors — it struck the bow section of the *Mont Blanc,* a French munitions vessel en route to the Basin to queue up for a transatlantic convoy. The collision occurred at the Narrows, the least wide portion of Halifax Harbour, where north Haligonians and their Dartmouth neighbours are almost within hailing distance. What would have been a minor collision was rendered lethal by the thousands of tons of highly explosive materials on board the French ship. The now burning *Mont Blanc* drifted towards the Richmond area of north Halifax, its crew having quickly vacated the ship. Hundreds of spectators lined the docks and windows along the waterfront, taking in the spectacle. Most of these perished in the blast which followed, powerful enough to hurl a 1,140-pound anchor two miles and to break windows fifty miles distant. The *Mont Blanc* disintegrated, its hull turned into deadly shrapnel, and its death knell was heard over two hundred miles away.

Eerily, the *Titanic's* identical twin, the *Olympic,* was at anchor in the Bedford Basin at this time. Looming in the smoke like a ghostly forerunner, she silently witnessed the death of over sixteen thousand people and the maiming of another nine thousand. Her sister White Star Liner had sunk five years earlier, in 1912, killing 1,522 people; ironically, the blast rocked not only the *Olympic* but also the graves of hundreds of the *Titanic's* dead, buried not far from ground zero in Halifax's Fairview Lawn Cemetery.

Witnesses described the blast from afar as resembling a huge mushroom cloud, and Robert Oppenheimer later would study the effects of the explosion in calculating the strength of the atomic bombs destined for Hiroshima and Nagasaki. Over two square miles of the city were flattened, and the harbour was emptied of water, the subsequent tidal wave swamping the Dartmouth side and amplifying the toll of death and destruction. A black cloud hung over the city, and a toxic rain of tar and shrapnel fell for some time after.

Into this nightmare landscape were to arrive the first relief workers: a trainload of doctors, nurses and aid workers dispatched from the nearby communities of Kentville and Windsor. Among them was Dr. Percy McGrath, a recent graduate of Dalhousie Medical College, and his wife, a nurse. Unfortunately the railroad tracks were wrecked well out of the city, at Rockingham, and the rescuers had to trudge through rubble and past bodies "stacked like cord wood," on either side of their path. One doctor compared the flames and death all around to the nether regions of hell from Dante's *Inferno*.

Many of the injured were in horrific shape because flying glass had lacerated faces and damaged eyes. This was compounded by the fact that the sound of the blast had preceded the shock wave, luring many to run to their windows to see what happened seconds before the glass dissolved into a spray of razor-like shards. Conversely, the noise may have saved the life of the father-in-law of one of my patients. Mr. Robert Parker told me that his wife's father was driving a wagon just mounting the crest of a hill overlooking the *Mont Blanc* at the moment of detonation. The horse bolted at the sound and pulled the wagon around to the lee side of the hill, allowing the blast to pass over the driver's head without harming him.

Dorothea "Dot" Buchanan, a still-spry nonagenarian, related to me her experience of the explosion as a child of eight, living not far from the detonation site. Her family's grocery business was almost flattened, and a

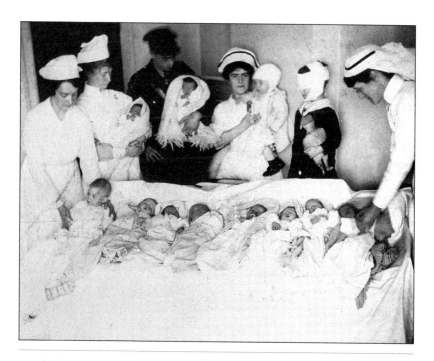

In the devastation of the Halifax Explosion, many babies were orphaned or separated from their families. They were gathered by rescuers from the wreckage of their homes and taken to hospital nurseries. KITZ COLLECTION, MARITIME MUSEUM OF THE ATLANTIC

large chunk of metal from the *Mont Blanc* fell though four levels of their large house, embedding itself in the cellar. The family lived in the walk-in meat locker of the grocery store for some time after. Dot's father, a tram driver, usually drove the waterfront route in Halifax, but due to the sickness of another driver he was doing the far-off Armdale route that day. The substitute driver on the waterfront route and the trolley car itself disappeared without a trace. The explosion blew the clothing right off many people, frequently without seriously injuring the nude victim. Dot recounts how her father happened on a woman naked in the street save for a purse and high heels. He garbed her in his coat, an act of generosity compounded by the fact that he also inadvertently gave her the trolley fares for the day, sixty-five dollars, in the garment's pocket, a small fortune in 1917.

Dot's family was luckier than most, with no serious losses. Many were less fortunate. An enumeration of common injuries suffered during the explosion included amputations, burns, lacerations and fractures as well as eye trauma. Thirty-seven people were left blinded and two hundred and six individuals lost an eye. The faces of many would remain disfigured throughout their lives. Incredibly, some victims, such as Barbara Orr, reported being pushed by the blast for a quarter of a mile without lethal injury. In the hard-hit Richmond area of the city, entire households were obliterated. There were many orphans, and the pitiful remnants of once-large families rejoined to mourn and bury their dead.

Initial relief efforts were hampered by fears that a second explosion would ensue from the munitions depot at the Wellington Barracks. Aid workers were forced to evacuate, leaving many to their fates in burning buildings. Records of the Halifax Children's Hospital, however, show that upon being ordered to clear the building, the feisty superintendent, blood dribbling down her face, declared, "No one shall leave this building. It would mean the death of many of the children if they had to be moved . . ., and if it should be that we are to die . . . it will be at our post." The Wellington munitions depot did not explode, thanks to the heroic efforts of Lieutenant C.A. McLennan, who doused hot coals blown into the bunker with a fire extinguisher. Another hero of the day was Vince Coleman, a worker at the Richmond railway yards, who stayed at his telegrapher's station to warn away trains advancing to their doom. He died instantly in the blast.

Needless to say, hospitals and morgues were overwhelmed by the gigantic load placed upon them. There were only four public hospitals in the Halifax area. The two largest were the Victoria General Hospital and the Nova Scotia Hospital for Infectious Disease, with less than four hundred beds between them, many already full. There was also the Children's Hospital and another tiny infectious disease clinic. Four military hospitals and seven smaller privately run facilities were also able to accept patients. An American hospital ship, the U.S.S. *Old Colony,* took on two hundred wounded. Though the Camp Hill military hospital had two hundred and eighty beds, it had fourteen hundred patients crammed into its wards and

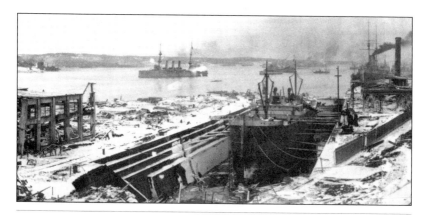

The morning after the Halifax Explosion. NATIONAL ARCHIVES OF CANADA, C-019953

corridors on December 6. Supplies of anaesthetics were limited, forcing many surgical procedures to be done without chloroform. Perhaps because many were still in shock, this did not present as much of an obstacle to surgery as might be expected. Supplies of anti-tetanus serum were also limited and were used only on very high risk injuries, but tetanus was rare and far less problematic than tuberculosis. Worsened by the cold, poor nutrition and crowded living conditions, the "White Plague" was soon stalking the corridors of the hospitals and the shelters for the displaced.

To compound matters, nature played a cruel joke by dumping sixteen inches of snow on the devastated city the day after the explosion. It was the worst blizzard in years and very unusual for Halifax at this season. There was a critical shortage of food, bedding and clothing. Clothes distribution was hampered by the reluctance of many with dead family members to wear colours other than black. The disruption of communications hampered the dissemination of news of the disaster, but once word had spread, aid poured in from all over Canada, including almost every town in Nova Scotia. The state of Massachusetts proved amazingly generous and contributed more than $750,000 in money and goods, a tremendous amount at that time. A train was dispatched from Boston carrying a team of thirteen physicians, as well as nurses, aid workers and some supplies. In appreciation of the state's efforts, the government of Nova Scotia each year donates a huge Christmas tree which graces Prudential Plaza in Boston.

Things gradually returned to some semblance of normality, though the rebuilding of the city, and more importantly, the lives of its citizens, would take many years. Many victims of the explosion would have suffered from what we today call Post-traumatic Stress Disorder (PTSD). An insightful American neurologist, Dr. William McDonald, warned other health care workers that survivors often needed treatment for emotional trauma as much as for physical injury. Without therapy, PTSD sufferers are often doomed to a life of anxiety, nightmares and obsessive fear.

The Halifax Relief Commission was formed to provide support to survivors. As recently as 1989, thirty people were still receiving benefits from its fund, though the commission itself was dismantled in 1975. In 1984, a monument to the victims of the Halifax Explosion, the Memorial Bell Tower, was inaugurated on the hill at Fort Needham in the north end of Halifax. The structure, reminiscent of the silhouette of a damaged building, incorporates a carillon of bells and was dedicated as a memorial the following summer, almost sixty-eight years after the explosion. Barbara (Orr) Thompson turned the sod for the ceremony at a site not far from where she'd been blown by the blast. Also present was nonagenarian Dr. Percy McGrath, travelling once more from Kentville as he had done many years before.

And who was to blame for the disaster? Rumours of sabotage by the Germans abounded but were dismissed. Initially the *Mont Blanc* was declared to be totally at fault, but ultimately the Supreme Court of Canada declared that each of the involved vessels was equally to blame. Regardless of who was at fault, every December 6 at nine a.m. a memorial service is held at Fort Needham in memory of the explosion's many victims. And on the hour, the sounds of the carillon bells ring out over Halifax's north end, floating across the Narrows to Dartmouth to remind all of this great tragedy.

George Burden

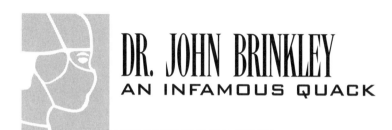

DR. JOHN BRINKLEY
AN INFAMOUS QUACK

"Say Au Revoir — but Not Goodbye," stated the front page of the Liverpool paper when Dr. John Brinkley's hundred-and-ten-foot yacht left the harbour in August of 1936.

Everyone in the small community was in awe of the American millionaire. That year, he had invited the mayor and town councillors and their wives on board his yacht, where he entertained them lavishly. And, although little was known about the man, his ostentatious lifestyle and his exceptional fishing skills had greatly impressed the townspeople. Everybody knew that Brinkley had set a new record by landing a three-hundred-and-sixty-kilogram tuna, and he had told them that he was a physician practising in Del Rio, Texas.

Years later, local historian Armand Wigglesworth, who was a young boy when he met him during one of Brinkley's visits to Liverpool, mentions this intriguing fellow in his book, *Anecdotes of Queens County, Nova Scotia* (Volume 2). He writes that Dr. Brinkley always created a stir when he arrived on his magnificent yacht and reports that the doctor was reputed to have something to do with "monkey glands. A fertility scam, it was said."

Wigglesworth was mistaken about the monkey glands. It was goat testicles that, in the 1920s and 1930s, helped make John Brinkley one of the richest fraud artists in the United States. Brinkley's story is truly bizarre; the scams he perpetrated so successfully were so outrageous that it defies logic to think he managed to get away with them for more than twenty years.

John Romulus Brinkley was born in 1885. Where he was born is debatable; whenever he applied for a medical licence, he provided different birthplaces: Kentucky, Tennessee and North Carolina. What we do know about this charismatic man is that he attended what were then known as

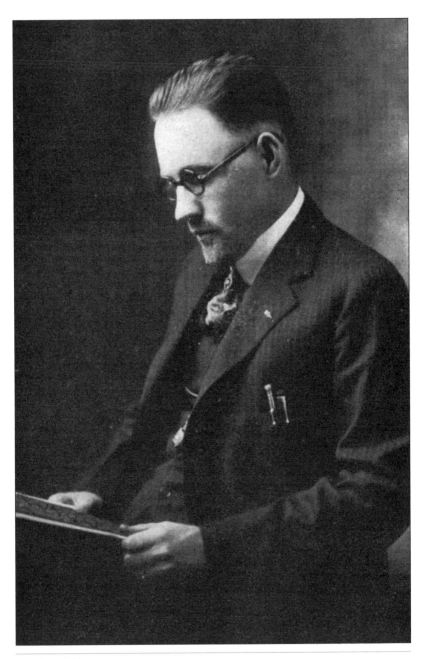

Dr. John Brinkley. *THE BRINKLEY OPERATION*

"eclectic" medical schools but never earned a legitimate medical degree. History has now revealed that two of the medical diplomas he displayed prominently on his office walls were purchased for about two hundred dollars each.

In 1917, after a brief time in the military — his army record indicates that he served as a medical officer for a little more than a month — Brinkley opened a medical office in an empty drugstore in Milford, Kansas. Unbelievably, though he had little formal medical training, he was soon actively involved in a general practice and treated people afflicted with a variety of common maladies.

A farmer known as "Mr. X" is said to have been the first patient to undergo Brinkley's innovative new therapy. The poor fellow visited the doctor secretly to express concern about his dramatically diminished libido. During their conversation, Brinkley jokingly commented that the man would not have any problem if had a pair of "those buck goat's glands in him." The farmer must have visualized the sexual stamina of his own goats and was captivated by such an exciting possibility. He implored the doctor to "put them in."

At first Brinkley had misgivings about performing this surgery, but then he relented, saying he felt compelled to help a patient who was desperate to find a medical solution for his "sagging" sex drive. Using a local anaesthetic, Brinkley carried out the strange procedure. He inserted a pair of testicles from a Tottenburg goat into the anatomically correct area of the man's body. Brinkley was delighted when later he learned that the goat testicles the farmer now possessed had, according to him, greatly enhanced his sex life. Even more remarkably, a year later, the man's wife is said to have given birth to a baby boy who was most appropriately named Billy.

After performing a number of his goat-gland transplant operations, Brinkley realized that he had discovered a way to make a great deal of money. He began to promote the surgery, mainly by gathering testimonials from grateful men who were willing to pay as much as a thousand dollars to regain their lost virility.

In 1918, buoyed by his success, Brinkley built a hospital where a number of patients could be treated. One of his marketing ploys was to offer prospective patients the unique privilege of choosing the goat that was to be sacrificed for their testicular implantation. To give his hospital more credibility, Brinkley also had a photograph of the Mayo Clinic hanging on his office wall. He began to describe himself as the hospital's Chief Surgeon, and he added M.D.C.M., Fellow of the American Association for the Advancement of Science and other credentials after his name.

News of Brinkley's phenomenal treatment was soon finding its way into the major newspapers. But when high-profile physicians were asked to comment on the goat-gland surgery, they invariably branded it as being entirely unsupported by scientific evidence. They also warned that it was potentially dangerous, and a number of deaths may have been linked to the procedure. One of Brinkley's most vocal critics was Dr. Morris Fishbein, the editor of the *Journal of the American Medical Association*. For many years, Fishbein wrote scathing articles about the man, whom he considered to be a quack. Brinkley hated him, and often he accused the American Medical Association of being intent on destroying an "outstanding pioneer in medical research." Some of Brinkley's loyal fans insisted that his achievements were in the same league as those of Louis Pasteur, the famous French chemist.

Amazingly, although there was growing opposition to his grotesque therapy, Brinkley's practice flourished. He began to give regular "health talks" on KFKB, Milford's radio station, which he just happened to own. Listeners as far away as Ontario could tune in to his "gland lectures," and apparently a few Canadians made the long trip to his hospital.

Always a brilliant entrepreneur, Brinkley recognized that it would be foolhardy for him to rely on making his goat-gland surgery the sole source of his income. He began to focus on other "male problems," including offering a "guaranteed" prostate treatment. But when he came up with the idea of radio consultations, he really hit the jackpot. Both his popularity and his income began to skyrocket. With the cooperation of several hundred greedy druggists, he was soon prescribing huge numbers of his mail-order prescriptions and earning as much as ten thousand dollars a week.

In the mid-1930s, when he was making regular summer cruises to the Atlantic region, Brinkley was a very rich man. American family doctors around the same period were earning an average of thirty-five hundred dollars a year, and specialists had yearly incomes of about seven thousand

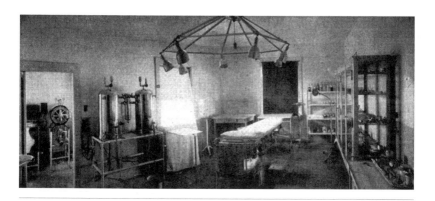

The operating room, Brinkley Hospital, Milford, Kansas. *THE BRINKLEY OPERATION*

dollars. Brinkley's estimated income in 1937 was a million dollars. But his crooked ways were bound to catch up with him, and when he became aware of the possibility of serious legal problems, he decided to leave Kansas and move to Del Rio, Texas, where he built himself a magnificent mansion. In his palatial new home he hung a huge photograph of himself wearing the uniform — unbelievably — of an admiral in the Kansas navy.

It is understandable that the residents of Liverpool were swept away by this charming man and his lavish lifestyle. The diamond watch and tie pins he liked to wear certainly helped create the fabulous image he loved to convey, as did the twenty-one-man crew who served on his yacht and had "Dr. Brinkley" emblazoned on their uniforms. As well, he liked to boast about the Lockheed Electra airplane he owned (which was eventually sold and used by the Royal Canadian Air Force for training purposes). Yes, the American millionaire yachtsman captivated the townsfolk of the seaside community.

One might have expected Brinkley to be smart enough to save some of his accumulated wealth and to give up his medical chicanery. He might then have been able to retreat quietly to his Texas estate to enjoy a tranquil retirement. But that did not happen.

In his excellent book, *The Roguish World of Doctor Brinkley*, author Gerald Carson provides an engrossing chronicle of this man's extraordinary life and untimely death. Carson reports that Brinkley died of a heart attack on March 26, 1942. Only fifty-six years old, he had been forced to declare bankruptcy and was facing a serious complaint filed by the United States Post Office. The complaint alleged that he was using the mails to "defraud in connection with his goat-gland treatment." It also stated that he and his group "did falsely pretend that John Brinkley was a great surgeon, scientist and physician, and that he, while visiting medical centres in Europe, had found a substance which would restore to normal sex vigour sexually weak men and women, and that the Brinkley treatment would cause men and women to live to be one hundred years old."

No doubt Brinkley was an outright con man, but he was also an astute businessman. Long before the advent of Viagra, he cleverly exploited a human frailty and made millions by misleading thousands of people. His claim, that he had found the secret to rekindling a man's sex life, was universally appealing. Carson laments that it is most unfortunate that Brinkley didn't direct his abilities towards more legitimate goals. He suggests that he might then have made a significant contribution to the field of medicine.

Brinkley certainly did make an intriguing contribution to a small town's history. He left behind memories of a dapper and charming American who was leading a life that the local residents could only envy. No wonder the Liverpool newspaper would bid him a fond farewell when his yacht departed the harbour. On these momentous occasions, the owners of fishing schooners and many small boats would show their respect by blowing their vessels' horns to wish him bon voyage, thus saluting one of North America's most notorious and successful charlatans.

Dorothy Grant

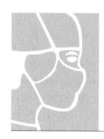

DR. ROBERT WRIGHT

SNOWMOBILE PIONEER

It was a cold January day in 1942, and the snow whirled and blew outside the windows of the old farmstead in Kennetcook. A four-year-old boy whimpered in his mother's arms as she sponged off the thin trickle of pus that oozed from her son's left ear. His temperature was high, and the loud crying of hours earlier had turned to ominous silence. His mother had called for Dr. Wright hours earlier, but nothing could move over the four-foot drifts that had buried all the roadways. Suddenly she saw a flicker of light in the field. Fatigue must be playing tricks on her eyes. Then she thought she heard a low droning noise like an airplane engine, but none of the aircraft at the nearby air base would be in the sky in weather like this. Then she saw it, a rooster plume of snow in the back field, thrown up by a strange propeller-driven vehicle, the weirdest contraption ever to grace her farm. It glided in past the old weathered barn and through the rickety front gate. An overcoat-clad figure, black bag in hand, rose and strode toward the front door of the farmhouse. The doctor had arrived. Dr. Wright quickly diagnosed the little boy as having mastoiditis, a serious infection of the bone behind the ear, and he drained the infected mastoid cavity right there on the old pine kitchen table. The child would make it, thanks to Dr. Wright and his mechanical sleigh.

Though no relation to Orville and Wilbur Wright, Dr. Robert Wright nevertheless deserves a place in the annals of transportation history. It all began in 1940, when he was a young family doctor fresh out of Dalhousie Medical School. Robert Wright and his wife Ritta settled in the little hamlet of Noel. Located on the shore of the Bay of Fundy, the town was originally an Acadian village dating from the 1700s. Founded in late December, it had been poetically dubbed Noel in honour of Christmas.

The local people, glad to see a new medic in the neighbourhood, welcomed the young couple with open arms. Dr. Annie Hennigar, one of the era's few female practitioners, was especially glad to see Robert so that she could cut back on her gruelling hours. She told him that he was welcome to do everything he wanted except pull teeth. That was to remain her domain.

The 1940s were the golden age of the medical house call, and Robert's practice covered a large geographic area. Furthermore, Noel and the surrounding communities were widely spread up and down the Fundy coast. Included in Dr. Wright's new domain was the County Home in Maitland, twenty miles from his dwelling, a daunting distance in these days. Among the forms of transportation the doctor used were a horse and buggy and a battered, but still serviceable, Model T Ford. Parts were scarce, there being a war on, but somehow Guy and Hollis Blackburn, mechanical geniuses and owners of the local service station, kept the car on the road.

The winter of 1940-1941 proved to be a hard one, with huge snowdrifts and nearly impossible travelling conditions. Fortunately, the Highway Department had introduced something which had never before graced the shore road: a snowplow. On its maiden voyage, the plow wended its way westward. Party lines hummed as people called family and friends giving a minute-by-minute rundown on the vehicle's exact locale. No one wanted to miss this feat of human ingenuity as it cut a swath through blizzard-blanketed roadways. Robert and Ritta received a breathless call that the plow would arrive any minute. When it did, they noticed with disappointment that it was riding on top of the drifts, leaving the road little if any clearer behind than in front, and gradually it was bogging down in the increasingly heavy snow. The Blackburn boys finally hauled the plow into their garage to see what they could do, but even their skills were not up to making the contraption snow-worthy. It took a week and nine men with shovels to get the vehicle the nine miles back to where it belonged.

Robert was no further ahead with his winter-travel dilemma until one of the Blackburn boys had a brilliant idea. Using two-inch copper plumbing pipe, the duo constructed a frame and mounted it on four skis crafted by Steve Hennigar, who was a master woodworker as well as Dr. Annie's brother. A Model A engine was mounted securely on the back, and a seat, steering gear, windscreen and headlight were bolted into place on the chassis. For the *pièce de résistance*, Steve Hennigar had made a wooden

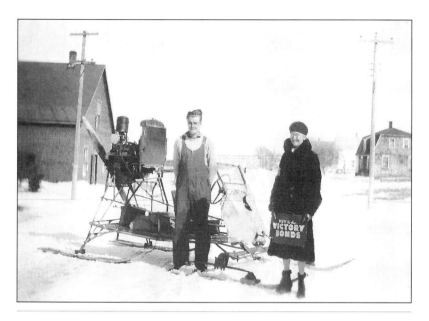

Dr. Robert Wright's snow plane, with designer Hollis Blackburn (left) and Pearl O'Brien (right), in 1941. When Dr. Wright wasn't using it, the propellor-driven vehicle was used to sell World War II Victory Bonds. ROBERT AND RITTA WRIGHT

propeller, and this was attached at the rear end of the Model A power plant. The engine started, and Steve's prop proved to be perfectly balanced, a neat achievement with a hand lathe. Thus was born the first snowmobile these parts had seen.

Robert found this to be just the ticket for his winter wanderings. His visits had to be mainly at nighttime so that the skis wouldn't stick in sun-melted snow. Townsfolk would often accompany him on his nightly forays, a cold ride for the rear passenger who lacked even the rude shelter provided the driver by the windshield. An instrument which was more valuable than any of his medical tools was the pair of wire cutters he used when the "snow plane," as they called it, had to travel cross-country over wire-fenced fields. Robert left a path of demolished fences behind him on his excursions, but never a complaint was heard from the local farmers, who knew it could be their families who might next need medical attention. An annoying glitch was that on bumps the propeller had a tendency to hit the rear skis and break, keeping Steve Hennigar busy at his lathe.

The sleigh proved to be a godsend to the community; many a baby was attended, many cases of pneumonia treated, and many an appendix removed before rupturing, thanks to its service. Among the memorable calls in the mechanical sleigh, Robert particularly remembers the night he arrived at an isolated dairy farm. As he passed the neat red barn, he heard the cows loudly mooing. The farmer's wife was in labour, and when Dr. Wright entered the house, he found the prospective father looking very anxious. "Thank God you're here, Doc! I'll leave you to tend to the wife. Those cows need milkin' some bad." With that he hurried to the barn.

In October 1942, Dr. Wright pulled up stakes and moved to Elmsdale, a town on the banks of the Shubenacadie River about thirty miles from Noel. Here he practised until retiring at the age of seventy-eight after over fifty years of practice.

Other memorable house calls include one by speedboat over the storm-tossed waters of Grand Lake to the isolated estate of E.H. Horne, the founder of the Noranda Mines. Perhaps to compensate for years of driving a prosaic Model T, Robert later bought a Karman Ghia sports car to use for his home visits. Nights spent in the "snow plane" gliding across moonlit fields may also have had something to do with his later learning to fly an airplane. But among Dr. Robert Wright's many housecalls, none was made in a vehicle quite as exotic as the Blackburn boys' propeller-driven brainchild.

George Burden

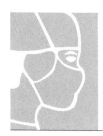

FERDINAND DEMARA
THE GREAT IMPOSTOR

When Dr. Joseph C. Cyr, a New Brunswick general practitioner, died in 2002, one of the obituaries written about him described him as the last surviving victim of a man whose incredible exploits inspired the 1960 movie *The Great Impostor*. Truth be known, Dr. Cyr was, in fact, only one of many individuals bamboozled by Ferdinand (Fred) Waldo Demara, an American who spent his entire life perpetrating numerous devious but brilliant hoaxes.

Dr. Cyr first meet Demara in Grand Falls, New Brunswick, in 1951, and at that time he was Brother John, a novice at a Trappist Monastery. The young physician would have found it hard to believe that this priestly fellow had a bizarre and infamous past. Since quitting high school, Demara had successfully passed himself off as a Doctor of Philosophy and a Doctor of Zoology; he had been a law student and a hospital orderly; and he had also spent time in the United States navy and army. (He had been court-martialled for going AWOL from the navy and spent eighteen months in a military jail.) Now in 1951, Demara was cleverly exploiting the mystique that his religious identity provided. This image was nothing new for him. At the age of sixteen, he had run away from home to join the Cistercian monks in Valley Fields, Rhode Island. A year later, he had transferred to the Brothers of Charity.

Brother John made a big impression on Dr. Cyr, especially when the monk revealed that, prior to joining his holy order, he been a physician. Dr. Cyr, who was a recent graduate of Laval University medical school, enjoyed discussing medical therapies with the monk and confided that he would like to obtain a licence to also practise in the United States. Years later, Demara said, "I told him that I would be only too glad to present

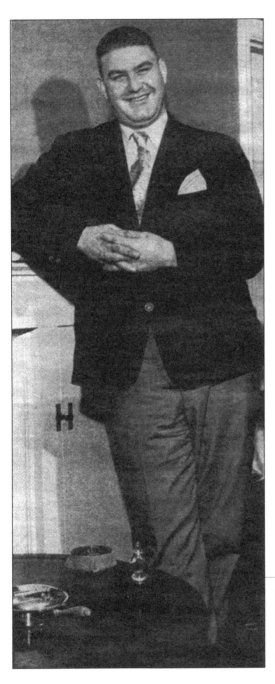

Ferdinand Demara,
photographed in his
parents' home soon
after he was discharged
from the Canadian Navy.
LIFE MAGAZINE

his credentials to the medical board in Maine. I didn't steal his papers. He gave them to me."

A few months later, Brother John, now calling himself Dr. Joseph Cyr, turned up at the Royal Canadian Navy recruiting depot in Saint John, New Brunswick. The petty officer on duty was ecstatic when the "physician" informed him that he wanted to serve overseas. The Korean War was underway, and the navy was desperate to sign up doctors. That evening "Dr. Cyr" was flown to Ottawa, where he received VIP treatment; his medical credentials were subjected to a cursory review at best. Within days he was commissioned a surgeon-lieutenant, fitted for new uniforms and assigned to duty at the navy hospital in Halifax.

There Demara exercised his deceptive powers. Whenever he encountered a serious illness, he consulted a senior medical officer, who was usually flattered that his colleague would seek his advice. He also came up with what he hoped was a foolproof treatment regime: anyone who had a sore throat or a bad cough was ritually treated with large doses of penicillin.

Ken Book, who now lives in Halifax, will never forget "Dr. Cyr." In the early 1950s, then a leading seaman in the navy, he developed painful blisters on his feet and, by chance, was seen by the "physician." "He looked at my feet and then gave me some papers to obtain white cotton socks. He also decided that I should get a shot of penicillin. I was about to leave his office when he advised me to come back to see him the following Monday. I told him that I would be going back to sea that day. When he heard this, he informed me that he would like to give me a second shot of penicillin, which he did."

Book says at the time he thought little of this unusual treatment, but then his condition changed dramatically. "I was staying with a friend for the weekend, and I soon developed swollen eyes and started to feel terrible. My friend got really worried and called an ambulance, which took me back to the hospital at Stadacona, where I stayed for several days. Turns out, I had a severe reaction to the penicillin, but I don't recall ever seeing Dr. Cyr again."

In 1962, I worked at the Canadian Forces Hospital on the Stadacona naval base in Halifax as a registered nurse. There I met a medical officer who had known "Dr. Cyr." He recalled a number of amusing incidents and told me the following story. One evening, he and his wife had invited "Dr. Cyr" to spend the evening with them. Their guest made quite an impression when he arrived carrying a dozen red roses, which he graciously presented to his hostess. The now-enlightened naval officer commented, "He really was a smooth character."

"Dr. Cyr's" credibility was finally questioned when he was transferred to the sick bay on the aircraft carrier HMCS *Magnificent*. Unable to hide his lack of medical knowledge, he performed poorly. The ship's commanding officer was not impressed, and in one of his reports he stated that "Cyr lacked training in medicine and surgery, especially diagnosis."

Despite this bad review, Demara's deception remained undiscovered, and he was soon re-assigned to HMCS *Cayuga*, a destroyer bound for Korea. On his first day on the ship, the imposter's medical skills were put to the test. Ordered to report to the captain's quarters, he found Commander James Plomer in agony, demanding that the "doctor" immediately extract an abscessed tooth. Excusing himself, Demara returned to his cabin, where he feverishly consulted his medical textbooks, something he often did. Equipped with a syringe full of Novocaine to dull his patient's pain, he returned to the captain's cabin, where he managed to yank out the offending tooth.

Demara's time in Korea would prove to be his undoing, not because of allegations of medical incompetence, but because of the stories that began to circulate about his superb surgical skills. It was soon being reported in Canadian newspapers that "Dr. Cyr," a brilliant navy surgeon, had performed many operations and amputations. Among these alleged accomplishments was a report that under extremely difficult conditions, he had performed successful chest surgery on a critically injured South Korean soldier. Demara later liked to claim that he had simply "read up" on that operation in *The Lancet*, the prestigious medical journal. No one really knows whether or not Demara actually performed any major surgery.

Demara did his best to stifle the unwanted publicity for the "life saving" surgery he had allegedly performed in Korea, but his "modesty" was to no avail. The navy's public relations staff could not afford to miss an opportunity to boast about their outstanding doctor and his extraordinary wartime achievements. Back in Canada, it seems that one of the people who read about the exploits of "Dr. Joseph Cyr" was none other

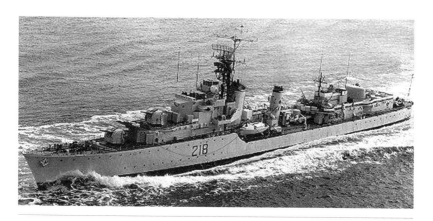

HMCS *Cayuga*, the ship on which Demara served. DND

than Mary Cyr, the real Dr. Cyr's mother. She contacted her son to let him know that a man on a Canadian navy ship in Korea was impersonating him, and the real Dr. Cyr immediately contacted the RCMP.

Commander Plomer, the captain of the *Cayuga*, was incredulous when he received a radio message: " We have information that Joseph C. Cyr, surgeon-lieutenant, 0-17669, is an impostor. Remove from active duty immediately, repeat immediately. Conduct investigation and report the facts to Chief of Naval Staff Ottawa." The commander thought this was a terrible mistake. He told "Joe" he was convinced that it was "a lot of rot," and ordered him to " carry on with your duty." Demara thanked him for his support, but a few days later he was ordered back to Canada. Rumour has it that he attempted suicide before returning to Canada, but individuals like Commander Plomer were convinced that this never happened.

To say the least, the Royal Canadian Navy was embarrassed that Demara had made fools of them. For some unexplained reason, they chose to let him off very lightly. They even granted him an honourable discharge, paid him the money he was owed and, it is believed, suggested "he leave the country." It has been alleged that the navy hadn't discovered that he wasn't a doctor, just that he wasn't the real Dr. Cyr.

Dr. Cyr and the Great Impostor did meet again when Dr. Cyr was a visiting physician at a hospital in California. Looking across an operating room, he was sure he recognized Demara, his face conveniently hidden behind a surgical mask. Demara was apparently working as a chaplain at the hospital, but Dr. Cyr choose not to "defrock" him.

For the last twenty years of his life, Demara continued to try brilliant though invariably implausible schemes. But it seems he could never recapture the excitement that he had once thrived on. A doctor who knew him during the final days called him "about the most miserable, unhappy man I have ever known." Ferdinand Waldo Demara was sixty when he died of a heart attack in 1982. Ironically, his ashes were scattered at sea.

Many of the people who knew him, especially his old navy buddies, remember him, not as a despicable con man, but as a true folk hero. The men on the *Cayuga* even sent their former shipmate a Christmas card from Korea. Enclosed in the card were some lines of verse written by one of the officers on the ship.

BECAUSE HE'S OUR FRIEND

He may be six kinds of a liar,
He may be ten kinds of a fool;
He may have faults that are dire,
And seem without reason or rule . . .
But we don't analyze, we just love him,
Because — well, because he's our friend.

Many of the men he served with in Korea actually admired Demara for his amazing ability to orchestrate a number of near-perfect "masquerades." No doubt he appreciated their admiration, and probably explained with a chuckle that what he had done had been prompted by what he liked to call "rascality, pure rascality!"

Dorothy Grant

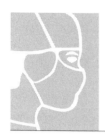

DR. R. ARNOLD BURDEN
SPRINGHILL RESCUER

I was digging at the coalface of the old Syndicate Mine in Springhill when the lights suddenly flashed out. Total darkness enveloped me, and for a second I panicked until I heard retired miner Blaine Hayden chuckling. He was our guide at the Miners' Museum in Springhill and was giving us a little taste of what trapped miners had experienced in past disasters. Except for the portion of the Syndicate Mine used by the museum, the mines in this small eastern Canadian community are now all closed. Although mining employed up to a thousand people at its peak, many are not sad to see the end of an industry that claimed the lives of over four hundred people through the years. The Syndicate Mine, shut down in 1970, was the last to close. Ironically, it claimed the life of the town's last mining victim when a resident working an illegal "bootleg" mine found himself emerging into the Syndicate's shaft. Sliding down a steep incline, he ran into a two-thousand-volt generator, and somehow his finger entered a minute hole, the only uninsulated portion of equipment. He was electrocuted.

Springhill has had three major mining disasters, explained Dr. R. Arnold Burden. Burden (not related to me) is a retired local family doctor who entered the mines to provide medical care during the last two. The first major disaster was the explosion of 1891, set off by an explosive charge used to loosen coal. One hundred and twenty-one people perished, including seventeen boys under seventeen years of age. The hero was young Danny Robertson, who, although badly burned himself, saved the life of twelve-year-old Willie Terris by carrying the child out of the pit to safety.

The explosion of 1956 was triggered by coal cars in the Number Two

Mine. On a cold night in January, the cars broke loose and slid down a steep incline, shearing a high-tension cable. The sparks ignited the highly inflammable coal dust. One of my own patients, John Pashkoski, was an eyewitness to the fireball that demolished the bankhead building, rising hundreds of feet into the air and killing five people on the surface.

Dr. Burden described how eerily masked draegermen — rescuers equipped with a breathing apparatus invented by Alexander Draeger — first entered the mine. Various toxic gases, which miners call "blackdamp," "whitedamp" and "afterdamp," filled the mine. Most deadly was "after-damp," or carbon monoxide, which is created after an explosion (hence the name). Following the draegermen came the "bare-faced" rescuers, including the doctor, who braved mine gases without protective gear. He had worked in the mines to help put himself through medical school and knew his way around as well as anyone. Dr. Burden noted that many of the victims showed the bright red lips of carbon monoxide poisoning. At one point he was overcome by gas himself and was briefly unconscious. Later a mine engineer by the name of Haslam approached Arnold Burden and showed him a note: "EVACUATE THE MINE WITH ALL POSSIBLE HASTE." Concentrations of explosive gas exceeding nineteen per cent had been detected. At twenty per cent the entire mine could explode, killing everyone in it, and the resulting fireball would kill many more at the surface. Fortunately the gases never quite reached this level.

The hero of the 1956 disaster was Deputy Overman Conrad "Con" Embree. Trapped with forty-six others and in danger of asphyxiation, he had the bright idea of cutting holes in a compressed air hose used to operate mine equipment. Hacking openings at one-foot intervals, each miner had enough fresh air to survive. Three of their number were dispatched to find help. This they did by "leapfrogging" up from one mine level to the next, tapping into compressed air at each interval. A lack of compressed air at the forty-six-hundred-foot level almost killed them. All told, thirty-nine men died and eighty-eight were rescued. This was to be neither the last nor the worst disaster the town would suffer before the end of the decade.

The Springhill "Bump" of October 23, 1958, rivetted world attention. Number Two Mine was one of the oldest and deepest in North America. When coal is removed from a seam, tension builds up in the hard rock

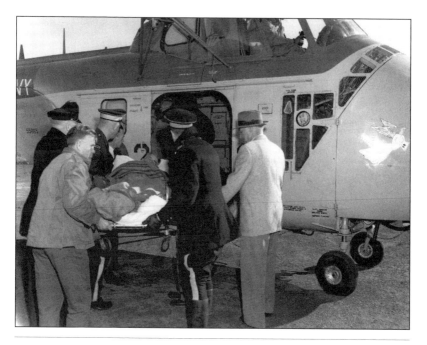

A helicopter evacuates a victim of the 1958 Springhill Bump, one of the worst mine disasters of the twentieth century. PUBLIC ARCHIVES OF NOVA SCOTIA

strata which overlie the mine, and the deeper the mine the greater the tension. Every once in a while this energy is released as an earthquake-like tremor called a "bump." Bumps were quite common at Springhill, especially in the Number Two Mine, and were usually quite mild. Not so this autumn evening. At 8:06 p.m. a massive bump occurred; it was felt over a fifteen-mile radius and registered on seismographs across eastern Canada. One hundred and seventy-four men were working in the mine. In many places the bump literally compressed the floor of the tunnel into the ceiling, and men were crushed like insects between two bricks. Arnold Burden told me that the locations of buried bodies were often identified by the trickle of blood oozing from between the collapsed areas of tunnels.

Once again Dr. Burden entered the disaster area. Luckily this time, in the absence of an explosion, there was no highly poisonous "afterdamp."

A trapped miner by the name of Leon Melanson was found partially buried. The leg of another miner was thought to be jammed under his chin, impeding rescue operations, and Dr. Burden was asked to amputate it. Arnold declined, and his suspicions were confirmed when subsequent digging revealed it was the man's own leg twisted into an "impossible" position by the force of the bump.

Other medical help came in the form of two young surgeons from Halifax. Dr. Charles Graham and Dr. Garth Vaughan flew in by military helicopter, bringing a load of drugs and supplies to assist the injured. Their landing field was the local ball field, lit by the headlights of cars belonging to the RCMP and the townsfolk. When they heard there were miners still trapped, they also entered the melee in the pit to render assistance.

Press coverage of "The Bump" was massive, and aid poured in amounting to millions of dollars. Hope of finding more survivors had just about been abandoned when world attention was again galvanized by the discovery of some men trapped at the thirteen-thousand-foot level. By chance a team of rescuers had walked past a broken six-inch pipe and heard a distant voice crying, "There are twelve of us in here!"

They were imprisoned behind eighty-three feet of solid coal and were suffering from hunger and dehydration. A smaller pipe was threaded through, and water and soup were pumped in. Rescuers took only fourteen hours to tunnel through to the trapped men, a task which normally would have taken several days. The last victims rescued were another group of seven, also at the thirteen-thousand-foot level. They had been reduced to drinking their own urine by the time they were freed, eight and a half days after "The Bump." One of these men, Maurice Ruddick, became known as the "The Singing Miner" when he told rescuers that if they gave him a drink, he'd sing them a song. A talented vocalist, he had been crooning to keep up the spirits of his fellows. The rescuers joked that Workmen's Compensation had sent them specially to find Maurice since the agency would be bankrupt if it had to look after his twelve children. One of his daughters, Sylvia, was once a patient of mine, and she, too, sings beautifully. Another miner told reporters he craved nothing so much as a 7-Up during his ordeal. The company sent him and the other miners a truckload of the beverage.

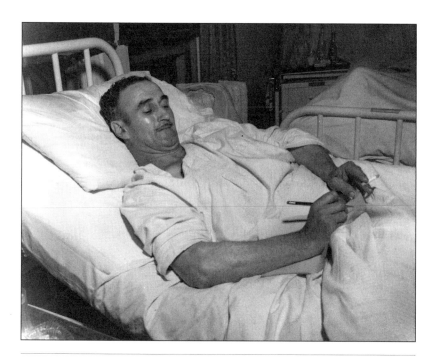

Maurice Ruddick, "The Singing Miner," enjoys a smoke in his hospital bed after his rescue from the pits. PUBLIC ARCHIVES OF NOVA SCOTIA

Many of the injured miners were admitted to Springhill's All Saints Hospital, and they were delighted when Prince Philip made a detour from an official visit to Ottawa to see them. Subsequently, Ed Sullivan invited Dr. Arnold Burden and two of the trapped miners, Gorley Kempt and Caleb Rushton, to be on his national television show. Less then twenty-four hours after leaving the mine, the exhausted trio found themselves in New York. They were gratified to see a Broadway theatre with the banner "More Men Alive" during the taxi ride to CBS studios. A bit worse for wear, they were loudly cheered by the audience when Sullivan introduced them. Springhill's rescuers were honoured with the Carnegie Medal for their courage, and the award now resides in the Springhill town hall. Dr. Burden later assisted the National Research Council of the Academy of

Sciences in Washington, D.C., in a disaster study entitled, "Individual and Group Behaviour in a Coal Mine Disaster," which was published in 1960.

With the end of coal mining, the town of Springhill found itself in dire economic straits. A minimum-security prison now provides some employment. More recently, superstar singer Anne Murray, a Springhill native, helped inaugurate an annual music festival. I had a chance to speak briefly with Ms. Murray, whose father, Dr. Carson Murray, had attended miners in hospital during and after the disaster. Anne, a physical education graduate before her singing career took off, also has two brothers who practise internal medicine in Maritime Canada.

Visitors to Springhill should be sure to take a tour of the Syndicate Mine to get a first-hand taste of the town's history. Despite a past marred by tragedy, the Springhillers remain a warm and welcoming people.

George Burden

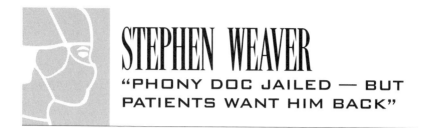

STEPHEN WEAVER

"PHONY DOC JAILED — BUT PATIENTS WANT HIM BACK"

Stephen Weaver's story is fascinating, not only because it involves an amazing con job, but also because of the public outcry that his masquerade provoked.

The tale began to unfold early in 1979, when Weaver, a thirty-four-year-old American, contacted Dr. M.R. MacDonald, the registrar of the Provincial Medical Board (PMB) in Nova Scotia. Identifying himself as "Dr. Stephen Weaver," he informed the registrar that he wished to discuss the possibility of establishing a medical practice in Lockeport. Weaver told Dr. MacDonald that he had recently been in touch with the Alberta Medical Association (AMA) and had learned that the small fishing community of seven hundred was in desperate need of a family doctor. He stated that he was anxious to be the physician who came to its rescue.

When questioned about his medical credentials, Weaver assured Dr. MacDonald that he had graduated from the University of North Dakota Medical School and had done a rotating internship at the University of Rochester Hospital in Minnesota. He also said that he held a Minnesota medical licence and certification from the National Board of Medical Examiners. Dr. MacDonald told "Dr." Weaver that his credentials appeared to be sound and added that there should be no reason why the young physician couldn't set up a family practice in town if he was able to meet the provincial medical board's criteria and satisfied the requirements of immigration authorities and Lockeport officials.

Dr. MacDonald apparently thought little more about that brief conversation until he began to hear about a young American doctor with a very busy medical practice in Lockeport, and disturbing calls began to arrive at the PMB office, requesting licensing information on the new physician.

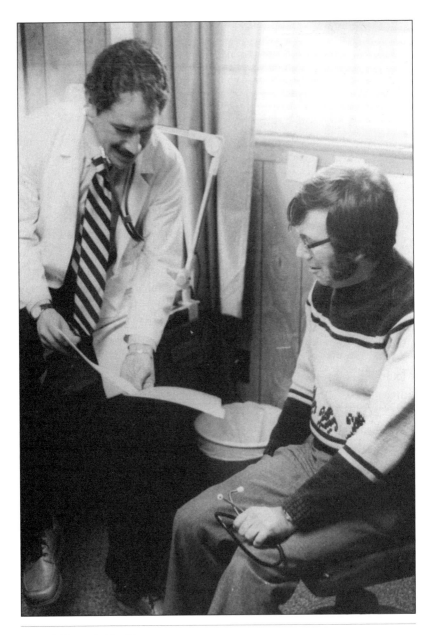

"Doc" Weaver in his office. SHELBURNE COUNTY MUSEUM

Dr. MacDonald, among a number of other observers, recognized that something strange was going on in the small South Shore community about two hundred kilometers from Halifax. In fact, the word bizarre probably best describes what was happening.

Just how Stephen Weaver managed to convince Lockeport town officials that he was a fully qualified physician with a licence to practice in Nova Scotia is not known. It appears that his debonair personality, smart grooming and good looks played a significant role in the deception. Dr. Stephen Woolf, a British physician who had come to Lockeport in February 1979, a short time before Weaver's arrival, found himself working closely with the town's other newcomer. Both men were daily seeing many patients, and it didn't take long before Dr. Woolf began to question Weaver's medical competence. "He saw all sorts of patients, mostly just routine work, but some quite serious," Woolf told a reporter later. "He was making a lot of mistakes, but nothing that made me think he was a fake."

Despite any medical shortcomings Weaver may have displayed, he convinced the administration staff at the Roseway Hospital in Shelburne, a town close to Lockeport, to grant him full privileges. This included the right to admit and treat patients, to assist in the operating room and to apply casts and suture wounds.

Weaver made a name for himself in the community within days of his arrival. His patients adored him and did everything to help his wife and two daughters adjust to a rural lifestyle. The pastor at one of the town's churches became one of many who viewed Weaver as a highly competent and dedicated physician. "Money wasn't his objective," the pastor said. "Dr. Weaver loved medicine, loved helping people."

Because he did not have a licence to practise medicine in Nova Scotia and therefore had no billing number, Weaver attempted to fund his illegal activities by charging his patients for only the percentage of medical payments not covered, at that time, by the province's health insurance plan, fifteen per cent of the total fee. This meagre compensation meant that he was earning only a couple of hundred dollars a week, although he was seeing a large number of patients every day. It was not enough money to cover his expenses, and, faced with the implications of his inadequate income, Weaver made a big mistake – he applied for provincial health insurance payments. At the same time, a pharmacist in Lockeport had become concerned about the appropriateness of his prescribing habits and was raising questions about Weaver's credibility. The investigations revealed that Weaver had never graduated from any medical school in the United States. There was further alarming evidence that he had also posed as a qualified physician while working at a clinic in a ghetto area of Washington, D.C.

Weaver's fraud came to an abrupt end on April 10, 1979. On that day, the RCMP arrived at his door and, under the Medical Act of Nova Scotia, formally charged him with practising medicine without a licence. They also charged him with criminal negligence, assault causing bodily harm and possession of the drug Demerol for purposes of trafficking.

News of Weaver's arrest created chaos in Lockeport. Less than twenty-four hours later, the mayor appeared on television to warn residents against taking any medications that had been prescribed by Dr. Weaver. Some panic-stricken townsfolk immediately threw their prescriptions down the drain and began to besiege the town pharmacist and Dr. Woolf, the sole remaining physician. They wanted someone to assure them that their lives were not endangered. Provincial newspapers headlined stories of the humiliating fiasco, and some of the patients who had been seeing Weaver began to experience an array of symptoms, including dizzy spells, headaches and nausea. One woman declared, "He's caused us a lot of trouble!"

But others who had been Weaver's patients didn't share this hysteria. They were furious that the mayor had created widespread fear by issuing a warning. They contended that his action was totally unwarranted, and many of them simply refused to believe that Weaver was not a qualified physician.

What these people did not know was that their hero's lack of medical expertise had been creating anxiety among the medical establishment in the area for some time. Dr. Woolf had grown very concerned about Weaver's performance, and not long before his arrest, he had reported an incident to Dr. Frank Markus, the county's only surgeon. Woolf had consulted Dr. Markus after learning that Weaver had informed one of his patients that he was suffering from bladder cancer when it was clear the man's symptoms were caused by a simple inguinal hernia. Drs. Woolf and Markus were planning to raise their concerns at a medical meeting to be held after the Easter holidays. The law mercifully intervened a few days before that could happen.

After his arrest, Weaver was incarcerated in the Shelburne County Jail. His wife, Sandi, who apparently had never doubted that her husband was a qualified physician, suddenly found herself destitute. Within twenty-four hours of her husband's arrest, the landlord advised her that he wanted the family out of their rented home. To make matters worse, a local bank froze her husband's account and seized his car. Left with only two dollars to her name, Sandi Weaver was devastated and felt totally abandoned. Fortunately, people in the close-knit community responded. They bought groceries, collected a thousand dollars and found a small cottage where she and her daughters could live.

Meanwhile, the jailed but unrepentant Weaver was telling his story to reporters and others. This dramatic episode in his life clearly revealed that he was a man with an enormous ego. Interviewed at the jail, only a short distance from the community of Lockeport where he had hung out his shingle, Weaver told a reporter, "From the point of book knowledge, I know more than most doctors. What I lacked was practical knowledge, and this I gained in Lockeport. I feel I am qualified."

According to Weaver, he was the son of a full-blood Comanche Indian father and an Irish-American mother. At the age of two, he said, he had been adopted by a Jacksonville, Florida, couple, and he received his early education in that state. Although an RCMP investigation failed to show that he had ever attended university, Weaver insisted that he had been enrolled at Jacksonville University, where, he claimed, he had often been on the dean's list. He also alleged that he had once earned $30,000 a year as a computer salesman, but that he had always dreamed of becoming a physician.

In an article that appeared in the June 21, 1979 issue of *The Barometer*, a now-defunct Halifax weekly, he told a reporter, "I chose to practise as a doctor because I feel I have an innate ability. This was not a spur of the moment decision. I prepared myself very carefully. I began by writing to the University of North Dakota's Medical School. I bought the required books and studied their curriculum. Having mastered all the theory, I had to find a way into practice." To put the theory that he claimed to have mastered into practice, he had contacted the Alberta Medical Association asking for rural medical vacancies, "specifically, places where no other doctors would want to go."

The secretary at the AMA who sent Weaver a list of rural vacancies had circled Lockeport and added a note in the margin advising him that the town had been looking for a doctor for more than two years. Weaver was only too happy to take advantage of the community's dilemma. Asked if he felt any remorse for his deception, Weaver replied, "Why should I? I lied to no one. I volunteered no information about myself, and I was never asked at any time if I was a doctor." When asked to explain how he could possibly defend the charade he had orchestrated, he replied, "In the two months that I practised in Lockeport, I learned more than most interns learn in a year in a hospital because I saw a wide range of ages and a variety of ailments. I saw eleven hundred people in that space of time. I'm glad I did it. It was a great experience, very enlightening."

When questioned about the wisdom of suturing patients when he had no medical training, Weaver told an interrogating RCMP officer that he had practised on grapefruit. Asked just how long he had expected to get away with the deception, Weaver, who reportedly had become more and more arrogant, said, "If I'd been the only doctor in Lockeport, as I'd expected to be, I could have gotten away with it indefinitely!"

On May 29, 1979, Stephen Weaver, who had pleaded guilty to practising medicine without a licence and to the charge of possessing the drug Demerol for the purpose of trafficking, had his final day in court. He received a five-hundred-dollar fine and a six-month jail sentence.

Everything about Weaver's short stay in Lockeport and his impact on the people in the small town was extraordinary. His charismatic personality was dramatically illustrated during the time he spent in the Shelburne County Jail. Other inmates were so impressed with his "performance" and the wonderful fiction he spun that they somehow managed to establish a bail fund for him.

Weaver's scam proved to be such titillating news that even the *National Enquirer* gave his escapades coverage in one of its June 1979 issues. He was still in jail when the tabloid ran a column featuring his picture with the caption, "'Doctor' Weaver treats a young patient while he was in the Canadian fishing village of Lockeport." The story was headlined "Phony doc is jailed – but his 'patients' want him back."

In mid-July of 1979, Weaver was released from prison and deported back to the United States. No one seems to know what happened to "Doc" Weaver, although he did tell friends that he had applied for admission to the University of Colorado Medical School.

Long after Weaver's ignominious departure, many of his supporters continued to believe that he was a real doctor. In a story featured in the *New York Star*, the pastor who had been one of his staunchest supporters told a reporter that if Stephen Weaver were to return to Nova Scotia, many Lockeport residents would see him again because "here was a man who really loved small-town folk, and the love he gave was returned in equal measure."

No doubt. "Doc" Weaver would not have been surprised in the least to learn of this display of lasting admiration for the brief but unforgettable time he had spent in the community. This vote of confidence would simply have justified his firmly held conviction that he had been "one of the best doctors" the town ever had.

Dorothy Grant

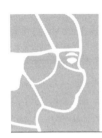

DOCTOR ON THE RUN

In late 1992, when the Yarmouth Regional Hospital successfully re-cruited Norris Jagnandan, a physician from the southern United States, staff members were jubilant. For years, the facility had been plagued with understaffing at its twenty-four-hour emergency and outpatient department. Desperate to find a general practitioner to help cover outpatient rotations, the hospital had first advertised across Canada and then in the United States. Only three physicians had responded.

When their first choice backed out, Dr. Jagnandan, a forty-three-year-old physician who appeared to have an impressive background in emergency medicine, was considered. Several of his references were contacted, and the hospital heard only glowing reports of his moral character and medical acumen.

Early in September 1992, Dr. Norris Jagnandan's name was entered into the Medical Register in Nova Scotia. A short time later, along with a Finnish woman identified as his wife, Tuula, he moved to Yarmouth, where he established a practice and obtained a mortgage to purchase a home with frontage on picturesque Lake Milo.

The story might well have ended here except for the fact that Dr. Jagnandan quickly developed a disturbing reputation. There were allegations that he was often rude to his patients and arrogant to the hospital nursing staff, and there was growing evidence that his medical skills were, to say the least, deficient. In December 1993, the hospital had acquired a long string of serious, documented complaints about his attitude and medical care, and he had failed to respond to a warning that his status was at considerable risk. Therefore, the hospital suspended Dr. Jagnandan's privileges. The same month, the hospital followed appropriate protocol by advising the Provincial Medical Board (PMB) of the punitive step it had taken.

At about the same time, another hospital in Nova Scotia had contacted the board seeking information on a certain Dr. Norris Jagnandan, who had applied for privileges at their institution. They were advised not to proceed with his application until the board had time to conduct a further examination. What that examination revealed could be the makings of a best-selling book; on January 26, 1994, the PMB revoked Dr. Jagnandan's licence to practise medicine in Nova Scotia.

Dr. Norris Rajkumar Jagnandan graduated from the University of Mississippi School of Medicine in 1980. Soon after graduation, he spent three years with a United States army health clinic. This chapter of his medical career came to an end in 1983 when he was the subject of a general court martial and subsequently lost his clinical privileges. In 1987, Dr. Jagnandan was again in trouble when he had to surrender his medical licence in North Carolina after that state's Medical Board became aware of his army court martial.

Barely two years had passed when Dr. Jagnandan was again the subject of an investigation. In 1989, his licence to practise medicine in Georgia was suspended for "unprofessional conduct." It was subsequently reinstated and then suspended again in December 1991 in relation to the inappropriate prescribing of drugs and other substances. Evidence was later produced that he had traded drugs or prescriptions for high-quality Scotch and, on one occasion, for a set of golf clubs. There were further allegations of sexually related professional misconduct. Dr. Jagnandan had little choice but to sign an agreement with the state medical board that, pending a hearing to investigate allegations of serious professional misconduct, he would not practise in that state. But the disgraced physician was already plotting a way out of his dilemma.

To avoid a possible jail sentence, he decided to beat a hasty retreat out of Georgia; a bench warrant was issued for his arrest. He cleverly orchestrated a flight to Canada, where he hoped he could avoid retribution from American authorities. In fact, not long after he was accused of participating in criminal activities, the doctor was practising in Yarmouth, where he believed his sordid past would never be discovered.

Immigration authorities have not been willing to discuss what avenues

Dr. Jagnandan used to gain entrance to Canada, but the doctor who was the PMB's acting registrar at the time did say that it appeared the physician's documentation met Nova Scotia's licensing standards, and no further verification was undertaken. The PMB, which has since become the College of Physicians and Surgeons of Nova Scotia, now has procedures in place to detect fraudulent documentation. It also checks the Federation of State Medical Boards discipline data bank, which discloses suspensions, loss of medical licences, court martials and other misdemeanors.

When Dr. Jagnandan's past finally caught up to him, considerable attention was given to the question of how he had managed to obtain a medical licence in Nova Scotia. It was learned that the letter of good standing that an American doctor must provide to the provincial licensing authority from the last state in which he or she had practised was, in Jagnandan's case, a forgery. It also became clear that he lied in his original application for licensure in Nova Scotia when asked if his medical licence (registration or certification) had ever been revoked or suspended.

Dr. Jagnandan's wife also left behind an unpleasant reminder of the couple's brief stay in Canada: an outstanding warrant for her arrest on an impaired driving charge. She was charged on November 5, 1993, after the car she was driving was involved in an early-morning accident on the Bedford Highway.

So what happened to Dr. Jagnandan once he could no longer avoid the implications of his disgraceful past? Soon after he lost his licence to practice in Nova Scotia, he was arrested in a cheap hotel in Pori, Finland. His wife, Tuula, was not with him. After spending time in a prison there, an extradition petition by American authorities resulted in his being deported back to the United States.

On December 7, 1994, in the Superior Court of Troup County, Georgia, Dr. Jagnandan was found guilty of unlawfully distributing, dispensing, delivering and selling controlled substances without a written or oral prescription and otherwise violating the Georgia Controlled Substances Act. The court noted that he continued to deny any criminal conduct and expressed no sense of remorse. He was sentenced to five years: a two-year prison term and three years' probation. He was also prohibited from practising medicine during the term of his sentence and fined $25,000 and his home and boat were seized by the state.

Immediately after his court appearance, Dr. Jagnandan was sent first to a Troup County jail and then to a Georgia state prison. He remained an inmate at the prison until he was paroled on January 11, 1996. But true to form, Dr. Jagnandan violated the terms of his parole and fled the state. On February 15, 1996, the state of Mississippi, based on what had taken place in Nova Scotia and Georgia, revoked Dr. Jagnandan's licence. On November 4, 1996, after numerous attempts to reach him were unsuccessful, the Georgia State Board of Medical Examiners also revoked his medical licence.

Pete Skandalakis, Troup County's district attorney, made it clear that he will never forget the infamous Dr. Norris Jagnandan. In a telephone interview, he described him as being "one of the most cunning, devious and self-centred people I have ever met." Skandalakis also disclosed that there is a violation of parole warrant pending for Dr. Jagnandan's arrest. "If we find him, he will be returned to prison immediately."

In the end, Dr. Jagnandan has pulled off yet another remarkable vanishing act. To date, there have been no further reports of where this illusive and unscrupulous man may be hiding.

Dorothy Grant

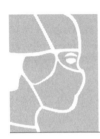

A TIME TO GRIEVE

During his more than thirty years as a pathologist, Dr. John Butt, who for several years was Nova Scotia's chief medical examiner, has had to deal with many tragedies, including a 1986 train crash in Alberta that killed twenty-three people. He says, however, that nothing ever came close to the heartbreaking tragedy of the crash of a Swissair flight that occurred on September 3, 1998, near Peggy's Cove in the Atlantic off Nova Scotia.

Butt still finds it difficult to describe his feelings the night Swissair Flight 111 went down close to his home in St. Margaret's Bay. "It seemed incredible to me because I've often watched international flights pass over my house." He vividly recalls trying to come to terms with the magnitude of the disaster that he and countless others now had to confront. "For one thing, we didn't have any kind of disaster plan to guide us through the horrors we were facing. And, even if we had had some material like that, nothing can ever prepare you for such a horrible event."

After throwing a few pieces of clothing into a suitcase, Dr. Butt went to Canadian Forces Base Shearwater, where a temporary morgue had been set up. A devastating scene awaited him. "Soldiers were taping the floor to receive bodies. There was yellow tape all over the place. Sadly, only a single body would ever come to rest on one of those taped areas." At first, there were reports of survivors, but optimism quickly vanished. "We were told that thirty-six or thirty-seven bodies had been recovered, but there was absolutely no basis to this information. I think I first comprehended the magnitude of the disaster when I went on a naval helicopter to HMCS *Preserver*, the mother ship of the recovery fleet. What I saw was beyond belief — there were basically only fragmented remains. At that

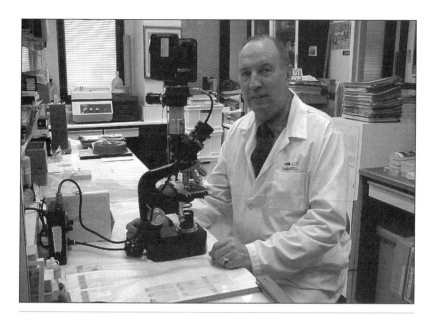

Dr. John C. Butt. COURTESY OF DR. JOHN C. BUTT

point I felt overwhelmed," says Dr. Butt, shaking his head. "It crossed my mind that the sailors were in a very unenviable position. God knows what happened to them, but, hopefully, they're working through it."

The next few days were numbing. "Conditions were terrible. I don't remember going to bed for many hours, as we were desperately working our way through the horrific process of identification. We did write some very tight guidelines for the use of DNA, but we had to modify them almost immediately, because we were overwhelmed with small material."

It was on Friday, three days after the crash, that Dr. Butt faced what he has called "the eye of the storm." With the president of Swissair and members of the RCMP, he sat on a platform in the ballroom of the Lord Nelson Hotel in Halifax and faced the hundreds of people who had lost someone on Flight 111. "While I was waiting to speak, I looked out into the audience and witnessed extraordinary pain. It was a huge experience. My throat was full of emotion, and I know my voice did quiver. I had to tell the awful truth to those people and be honest with myself. I couldn't turn myself back into some sort of a scientific parrot. At that point, I felt tremendous anguish because of what I knew I had to say: 'I regret that none of you will ever be able to see your family member again.' I remember one man in particular. I shall never forget the expression on his face. It was ghastly — dried out with grief."

One couple in the front row of the auditorium listened intently to the terrible news and then wistfully asked Dr. Butt if he had any knowledge of a black woman, a relative who had died on the flight. "This was amazing to me," the medical examiner says. "I asked them to come to see me after the meeting was over. A black woman's body had, in fact, been found, and her family was the only one able to make a visual identification."

Dr. Butt's face perceptibly changes as he recalls the end of the meeting, when he found himself surrounded by the crash victims' families. They must have sensed his vulnerability and compassion. "Some of them wanted to touch, hold or hug me. People reached out to shake my hand. One young man, who had expressed a lot of anger earlier, came up to speak with me. He was gracious as he introduced his mother, who said, 'I don't believe any of this, you know. None of this is true.' Our eyes met, and I held her hand." He pauses, reliving the intensity of that moment, "It was emotional beyond words," he says, his eyes tearful. "There was a transfer of energy. I truly believe at that moment she began to accept that something unspeakable had happened."

Like most pathologists, and indeed many physicians, Dr. Butt says that, in the past, it has often been possible for him to avoid dealing with the emotional trauma that is associated with the death of a loved one. He knows he has sometimes limited his exposure to the families who have lost someone under tragic circumstances. "I set up a barrier of sorts by either having a nurse act as an intermediary, or often by discussing such situations over the phone." His tone is suddenly emphatic. "I can't do that any more because it's selfish. I feel strongly that there is a great need to relate to families."

Dr. Butt speaks highly of the hundreds of dedicated people, many of them doctors, nurses and technicians, who faced the grisly task of helping to identify the shattered human remains that were retrieved from the depths of the Atlantic Ocean. He also admires the individuals who provided one-on-one support for grief-stricken men, women and children. But it is the families of the victims of Flight 111 who have earned his greatest respect.

"It was tough and a humbling experience. I have no strong connections with anyone other than the relatives. The nature of the human remains didn't permit that; there was nothing about them that was memorable in terms of catching a glimpse of the two hundred and twenty-nine individuals who died. I think it is only important to see things through the families' eyes. What I want to see happen is for the brutality and terror to fade, and there will be more memories of individuals. After all, isn't that what life is really all about?"

After being interviewed by dozens of media outlets during the months that followed the air disaster, Dr. Butt is clearly tired and emotionally drained. But he does not hesitate, when asked, to articulate the impact the plane crash had on him. "I don't consider myself to be a religious man, but the tragedy has opened a spiritual window for me." Asked about seeking closure, he responds with annoyance. "I don't want closure. In fact, I consider that word trite. What I want is a time to be alone, to reflect and occasionally to weep, to heal, and to come out of this great tragedy with the right kind of memories. For me, it was an amazing paradox that you can be working on something so awful and something good is going on at the same time."

He stops and appears to reflect on those harrowing yet rewarding days. "When we were working in that hangar, there was an enormous sense of direction — a sense of purpose. I never want to forget parts of that time in my life. What I do want most is more space, because I don't want to feel crowded by people talking about the disaster all the time. I want to talk about it, in my own time, to people I value and who will understand."

Dr. John Butt received the Order of Canada in the year 2000.

Dorothy Grant

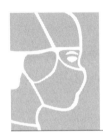

FURTHER READING

Bates, Walter. *The Mysterious Stranger*. Saint John: Geo. W. Day, 1887.

Bedwell, Stephen. "D'Anville's Doom: A Neurological Vignette from Historic Halifax," *Canadian Journal of Neurological Sciences* (February 1980).

Beed, Blair. *Titanic Victims in Halifax Graveyards / 2001*. Halifax: Dtours Visitors and Convention Service, 2001.

Blakely, Phyllis. *Nova Scotia's Two Remarkable Giants*. Windsor NS: Lancelot, 1970.

Brinkley, John R. *The Brinkley Operation*. Chicago: Sidney Flower, 1922.

Brown, Roger David. *Blood on the Coal: The Story of the Springhill Mining Disasters*. Hantsport NS: Lancelot, 1976.

Buckler, Helen. *Daniel Hale Williams: Negro Surgeon*. Toronto: Pittman, 1954.

Burden, Arnold and Andrew Safer. *Fifty Years of Emergencies*. Hantsport NS: Lancelot, 1991.

Carson, Gerald. *The Roguish World of Doctor Brinkley*. New York: Rinehart, 1960; Toronto: Clark, Irwin, 1960.

Cavin, Lee. *There Were Giants on the Earth*. Seville OH: Seville Chronicle, 1959.

Cramp, Arthur. *Nostrums and Quackery*. Vol. 3. Chicago: American Medical Association, 1936.

Crichton, Robert. *The Great Imposter*. New York: Random House, 1959.

Davie, Michael. *The Titanic: The Full Story of a Tragedy*. London: Grafton, 1987, 1996.

Dow, Leslie Smith. *Anna Leonowens: A Life Beyond* The King and I. Lawrencetown Beach NS: Pottersfield, 1991.

Elliott, James. "Obituary for Dr. Thomas 'Tam' Fyshe," *Hamilton Spectator* (October. 17, 1998).

Encyclopedia Titanica. http://www.encyclopedia-titanica.org.

Fishbein, Morris, M.D. *History of the American Medical Association*. Philadelphia: W.B. Saunders, 1947.

_____. "Modern Medical Charlatans," *Hygeia* (January 1938).

Grantmyre, Barbara. "Elmsdale 1785-1914," *Nova Scotia Historical Quarterly* (June 1972).

_____. *Lunar Rogue*. Fredericton: Brunswick, 1963.

Grosvenor, Edwin S. and Morgan Wesson. *Alexander Graham Bell: The Life and Times of the Man Who Invented the Telephone.* New York: Harry N. Abrams, 1997.

Hustak, Alan. *Titanic: The Canadian Story.* Montreal: Véhicule, 1998.

Kitz, Janet. *Shattered City: The Halifax Explosion and the Road to Recovery.* Halifax: Nimbus, 1989. Much of the material in "The Halifax Explosion: Taking Care of the Victims" comes from this excellent book.

Langille, Jacqueline. *Alexander Graham Bell.* Tantallon NS: Four East, 1989.

_____. *Giant Angus McAskill and Anna Swan.* Tantallon NS: Four East, 1990.

Lawson, Mrs. William. *History of the Townships of Dartmouth, Preston, Lawrencetown, Halifax County, Nova Scotia.* Halifax: Morton, 1893; facsimile reprint: Belleville ON: Mika Studio, 1972.

Lord, Walter. *A Night to Remember.* New York: Holt, Rinehart and Winston, 1955.

MacMillan, C. Lamont. *Memoirs of a Cape Breton Doctor.* Toronto: McGraw-Hill Ryerson, 1975.

MacNeil, Robert. *Burden of Desire.* Toronto: Harcourt, 1998.

Martin, John P. *The Story of Dartmouth (1886-1969).* Dartmouth NS: J. Martin, 1957.

McMillan, Beverly and Stanley Lehrer. *Titanic: Fortune and Fate.* New York: Simon and Shuster, 1998.

Maxtone-Graham, Joan, ed. *Titanic Survivor: The Newly Discovered Memoirs of Violet Jessop.* Dodds Ferry NY: Sheridan House, 1997.

Mitcham, Allison. *Prophet of the Wilderness: Abraham Gesner.* Hantsport NS: Lancelot, 1995. Much of the material in "Abraham Gesner: A Doctor Ahead of His Time" comes from this informative book.

Mowbray, Jay Henry. *Sinking of the Titanic: Eyewitness Accounts.* Mineola NY: Dover, 1998.

Nova Scotia Archives and Record Management, Halifax, Nova Scotia. Disposition of Bodies exTitanic, recovered up to May 13, 1912. List of bodies identified and disposition of same, list of bodies unidentified and disposition of same. Document D/S VK T53 D63 C4.

_____. "Preparations to Receive Bodies." *Titanic Commutator,* Spring 1983.

_____. Titanic, Record of Bodies and effects. Document VK 1255 T6 R35.

_____. "Woman Unknown," Inquest Report. 6 October, 1876.

Nunn, Bruce. *History with a Twist.* Halifax: Nimbus, 1998.

_____. *More History with a Twist.* Halifax: Nimbus, 2001.

Pritchard, James. *Anatomy of a Naval Disaster: The 1746 French Expedition to North America.* Montreal: McGill-Queens, 1995.

Raddall, Thomas. *Halifax, Warden of the North.* Toronto: McClelland and Stewart, 1971.

Ruffman, Alan. *Titanic Remembered: The Unsinkable Ship and Halifax.* Halifax: Formac, 1999.

Shephard, David A.E. "Alexander Graham Bell, Doctor of Medicine," *New England Journal of Medicine* (May 31, 1973).

Sherwood, Roland. *Legends, Oddities and Facts from the Maritime Provinces.* Hantsport NS: Lancelot, 1984.

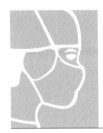

INDEX

A

Alexander Graham Bell Museum 61
American Museum 43, 44
American Revolution 16
Anderson, J.E. 16
Andrews, Tommy 65
Annapolis Royal, NS 14
Anville, Jean-Baptiste de la Rochefoucauld,
 Duc d' 12, 13-16
artificial lung 59, 61
Astor, John Jacob 70, 75-76
audiometer 59
Aylesford, NS 28

B

Baddeck, NS 59, 60, 61
Baldwin, Casey 61
Barbados 30, 32
Barnstead, John Henry 76
Barnum, Phineas T. 43, 44
Baron de Hirsch Jewish Cemetery 77
Bates, Captain Martin Van Buren 42, 44-46
Bates, Walter 24, 25, 26, 27
Beach, A.P. 45-46, 47
Bedwell, Stephen 16
Bell, Alexander Graham 57-61
Bell, Mabel (Hubbard) 57
Birch Cove, NS 14
Blackburn, Guy 92, 94
Blackburn, Hollis 92, 93, 94
Bond, Elizabeth 23
Bond, John 23
Book, Ken 97
Boston, MA 13, 14, 57, 83
Boyar, Avis (Fyshe) 56
Brantford, ON 57

Bras d'Or Lake, NS 58, 60
Brewe, Arthur 65, 69
Bridgetown, NS 41
Brinkley, John Romulus 85-90
Brother John. *See* Demara, Ferdinand Waldo
Buchanan, Dorothea "Dot" 80, 81, 82
Buckler, Helen 48, 52
Burden, R. Arnold 101-106
Butt, John C. 118-121

C

Cameron, Rev. John 38, 39-41
Canadian Forces Base Shearwater 118
Canadian Medical Corps 56
Cape Breton Island, NS 15, 34, 58, 61
Carpathia 69
Carson, Gerald 89-90
Cayuga 98, 99, 100
Ceylon 32
Charlottetown, PEI 20
Chicago, IL 48, 49, 51, 65, 79
Chulalongkorn, King 55
Civil War 44, 45
Cochrane, Rev. Rupert 44
Coleman, Vince 82
College of Physicians and Surgeons
 of Nova Scotia 116
Cornish, James 51
Cornwallis, Governor Edward 15
Cyr, Joseph 95, 97, 98, 99, 100
Cyr, Mary 99

D

Dartmouth, NS 79, 80, 84
Del Rio, TX 85, 87

Demara, Ferdinand Waldo 95-100
d'Estournelle, Vice Admiral 14
Dodge, Washington 65, 69
Draeger, Alexander 102
Duval, Lieutenant 14, 15, 16

E

East Hans Historical Museum 70
Edinburgh, Scotland 57
Elliott, Everett Edward 78
Elmsdale, NS 39, 41, 94
Embree, Conrad "Con" 102
England 16, 17, 31, 32, 36, 44, 65, 79
Englishtown, NS 35, 37
Eugenie, Empress 33

F

Fairview Lawn Cemetery 77, 80
Finn, W.D. 76
Fishbein, Morris 88
Fond du Lac, WI 65
Fortress Louisbourg 15
France 14
Frankfort, KY 65
Frauenthal, Henry 64, 68
Funeral Directors Association of the Maritime
    Provinces 71
Fyshe, Avis (Leonowens) 53, 55
Fyshe, James 53-56
Fyshe, Julia Corisande (Mattice) 55
Fyshe, Thomas 53, 55
Fyshe, Thomas "Tam" 55, 56

G

Garfield, James 58, 59, 60
Georges Island, NS 15
Gesner, Abraham 17-21
Gesner, Harriet (Webster) 17
Gilmour, George 56
Graham, Charles 104
Grand Falls, NB 95
Grand Lake, NS 94
Great Impostor, The 95

H

Halifax Explosion 79-84
Halifax, NS 13, 15, 16, 71, 73, 74, 75,
    76, 77, 78, 79-84, 97, 109, 111, 119
Halifax Relief Commission 84
Hamilton Club 49

Hamilton, ON 64, 68
Harper, Henry (Mrs.) 66
Harvey, Lt. Governor Sir John 20
Hayden, Blaine 101
Hennigar, Annie 92
Hennigar, Steve 92, 94
Horne, E.H. 94
hydrofoils 61

I

Imo 79
Ismay, Bruce 65

J

Jacksonville, FL 111
Jagnandan, Norris Rajkumar 114-117
Jagnandan, Tuula 114, 116
Jessop, Violet 66
John Snow & Sons 71, 72, 73
Jonquiere, Captain de la 14

K

Kempt, Gorley 105
Kennedy, Rev. James 28
Kennetcook, NS 91
Kentville, NS 78, 84
kerosene 19-20
Kingston, ON 24
Korean War 97, 98, 99, 100

L

Lake Loon, NS 28
Lake Milo, NS 114
Landon, Margaret 53
Lardner, Captain Fred 73
Leader, Alice 65, 69
Leonowens, Anna 53, 54, 55
Leonowens, Louis 54, 55
Lightoller, Charles H. 68
Lister, Joseph 49
Liverpool, NS 86, 89, 90
Lockeport, NS 107, 109, 110, 111, 112, 113
London, England 57
Louis XV, King 13, 14
Louisbourg, NS 15, 16
Lunar Rogue, The. *See* Moon, Henry
Lyell, Sir Charles 19

M

MacDonald, Dr. 59

MacDonald, M.R. 107
MacKay-Bennett 71, 72, 73, 74
MacKinnon, Clarence 78
Maitland, NS 92
Markus, Frank 110
Mayflower Curling Club 74, 76
McAskill, Angus 34, 35-37
McCurdy, John 60
McDonald, William 84
McGrath, Percy 80, 84
McKeen, Dr. 59
McLennan, Lieutenant C.A. 82
Melanson, Leon 104
metal detector 59, 60
Milford, KS 87, 88, 89
Millbrook, NS 43
Minahan, Lillian 65
Minahan, William 65, 68, 69
Minia 73
Mongkut, King 53
Mont Blanc 79, 80, 81, 84
Montreal, QC 74
Moon, Henry 22, 23-27
Moraweck, Ernest 65, 69
Mount Olivet Catholic Cemetery 77
Murray, Anne 106
Murray, Carson 106

N

Napoleon III 33
National Board of Medical Examiners 107
National Medical Foundation 51
New York, NY 13, 14, 51, 65, 66, 68, 69
Newell, A.W. 76
Newell, Frank 76
Nine Mile River, NS 39
Noel, NS 91, 94
North Sydney, NS 35
Northumberland, Le 15

O

O'Brien, Pearl 93
O'Loughlin, William 63-64, 65, 66, 67, 68
O'Neil, Annie 71
Olympic 79, 80
Oppenheimer, Robert 80
Ottawa, ON 97

P

Paddock, Adino, Jr. 24

Pain, Alfred 62, 64-65, 68
Palmer, Henry 49
Parker, Robert 80
Parrsboro, NS 17, 19
Pashkoski, John 102
Peace River, AB 56
Peggy's Cove, NS 118
Philadelphia, PA 39, 40, 65, 69
Philip, Prince 105
Pine Hill, NS 78
Plomer, Commander James 98, 99
Provincial Medical Board 107, 115
Public Archives of Nova Scotia 75

R

RCMP 99, 104, 110, 111, 112, 119
Rawdon, NS 23
Reynolds, Emma 49, 51
Reynolds, Rev. Louis 49
Richmond, NS 79, 82
Robb, James 19, 20
Robertson, Danny 101
Robinson, J.D. 46
Rockingham, NS 80
Royal Canadian Air Force 89
Royal Canadian Navy 96, 97, 99
Ruddick, Maurice 104, 105
Ruddick, Sylvia 104
Rushton, Caleb 105

S

Sable Island, NS 13
St. Ann's Bay 37
Saint John, NB 19, 71, 97
St. Margaret's Bay, NS 118
San Francisco, CA 65, 79
Scotland 16, 35
Selma, NS 70
Seville, OH 45
Shelburne, NS 109, 111, 112
Shubenacadie, NS 40
Shubenacadie River, NS 39, 94
Simpson, J. Edward 64, 66, 67, 68
Simpson, James 44
Skandalakis, Pete 117
Sleet, Jessie 51
Sloan, Mary 66, 67
Smith, Henry More. *See* Moon, Henry
Snow, John 72
snow plane 91-94

Springhill, NS 101-106
Springhill Miners' Museum 101
Stadacona Naval Base 97
Stuart, Charles (Bonnie Prince Charlie) 16
Sullivan, Ed 105
Swan, Anna 42, 43-47
Swan, Dale 46
Swissair Flight 111 118-121
Syndicate Mine 101, 106

T
telephone 57, 61
Terris, Willie 101
Thailand 53, 54, 55
Thompson, Barbara (Orr) 82, 84
Thompson, Catherine Ann 28-33
Thompson, Colonel George Forbes
    28-33
Thompson, Mary (Taylor) 28-33
Thumb, Colonel Tom 36
Titanic 62, 63-69, 70, 71, 74-78, 79, 80
Toronto, ON 21, 26
Troup County, GA 116
Truro, NS 43

U
United States 51, 52, 85, 95, 110, 113, 114

V
Vaughan, Garth 104
Victoria, Queen 36, 43, 44

W
W.W. Cole Circus 45
Walsh, Elizabeth 71
Walter, M., Rabbi 77
Washington, DC 50, 51, 57, 110
Waterhole, AB 56
Weaver, Sandi 111
Weaver, Stephen 107-113
Webster, Issac 17
Wellington Barracks 82
White Star Line 63, 65, 71, 72, 73, 74, 75
Wigglesworth, Armand 85
Williams, Daniel Hale 48-52
Windsor, NS 80
Woolf, Stephen 109, 110
World War I 61, 79
World War II 93
Wright, Ritta 91, 92

Wright, Robert 91-94

X
X-ray 58, 59, 61

Y
Yarmouth, NS 48, 76, 114, 115

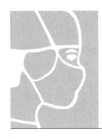

THE AUTHORS

my Doc.

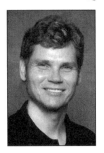

A native of Newfoundland, Dr. GEORGE BURDEN is a general practictioner in Elmsdale, Nova Scotia. His career as a medical historian began when he discovered that the early Roman emperors may have been afflicted by Tourette Syndrome. Encouraged by praise from Dr. Oliver Sacks and CBC Radio's *Quirks and Quarks*, he investigated ancient Egyptian medicine, and at the same time he discovered the treasure trove of medical history closer to home. His stories appear frequently in *The Medical Post* and *The Halifax Sunday Herald*, and he has contributed to *The St. John's Telegram, Stitches Magazine of Medical Humour* and *The Reader's Digest*.

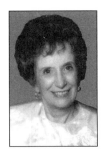

DOROTHY GRANT chose nursing as her first career, radio and television journalism as her second and working as the Medical Society of Nova Scotia's Director of Communications and Public Relations as her third. All the while, she nurtured an irrepressible passion for writing. She has published stories in periodicals including *The Canadian Medical Association Journal, Family Practice Magazine* and *The Pharmacy Post*. A frequent contributor to the Halifax *Chronicle-Herald* and *Sunday Herald*, she has contributed more than sixty articles to *The Medical Post*. Dorothy Grant lives in Hammonds Plains, Nova Scotia, just outside Halifax.